Cardiac Arrhythmias - Translational Approach from Pathophysiology to Advanced Care

Edited by Endre Zima

Published in London, United Kingdom

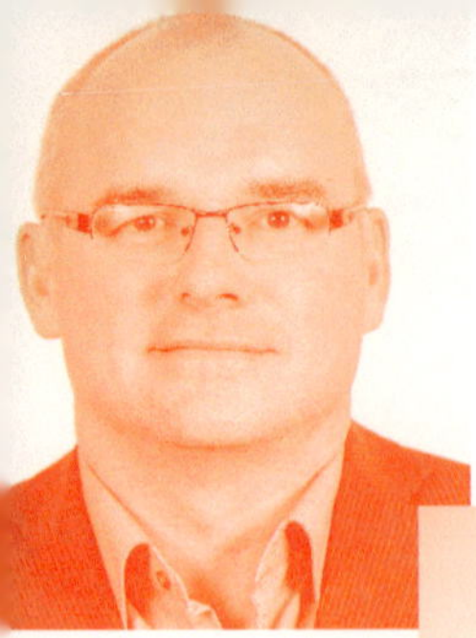
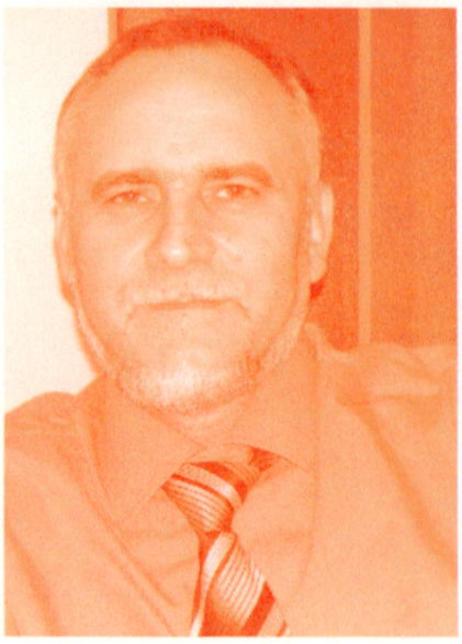
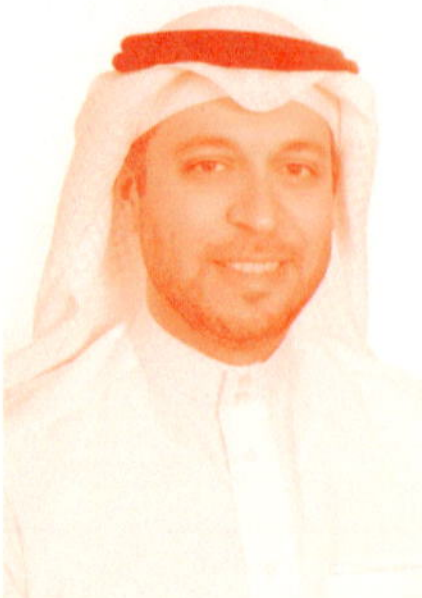
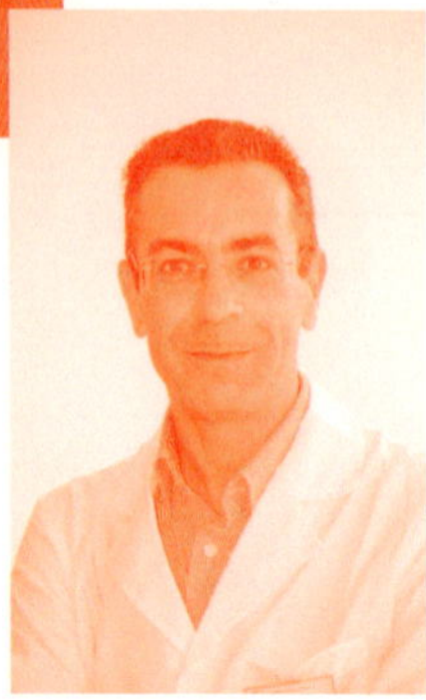
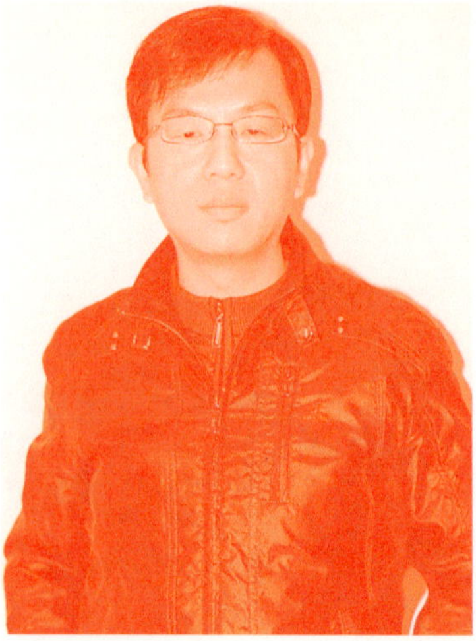
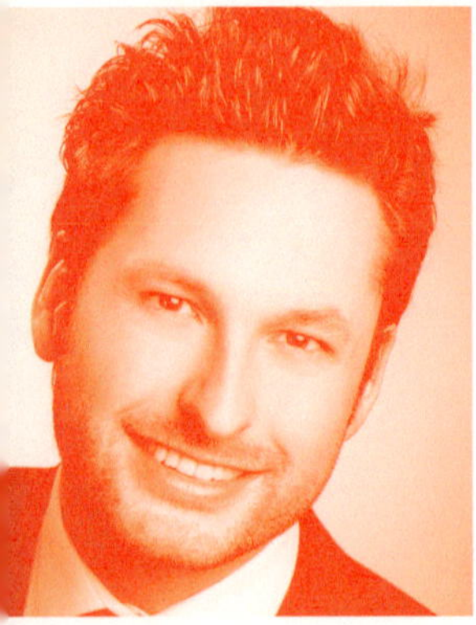
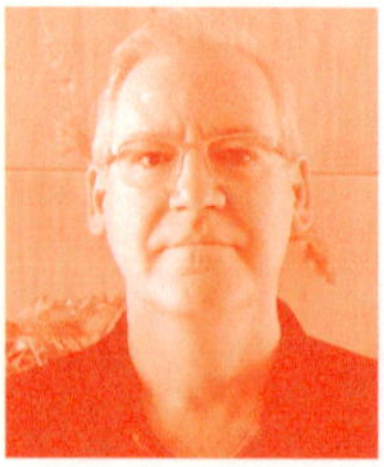

IntechOpen

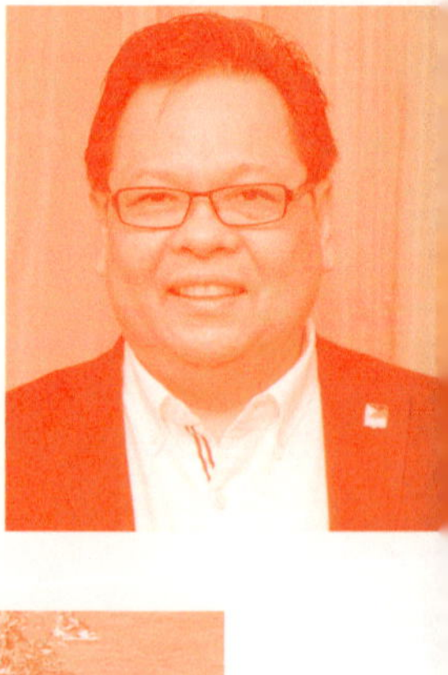
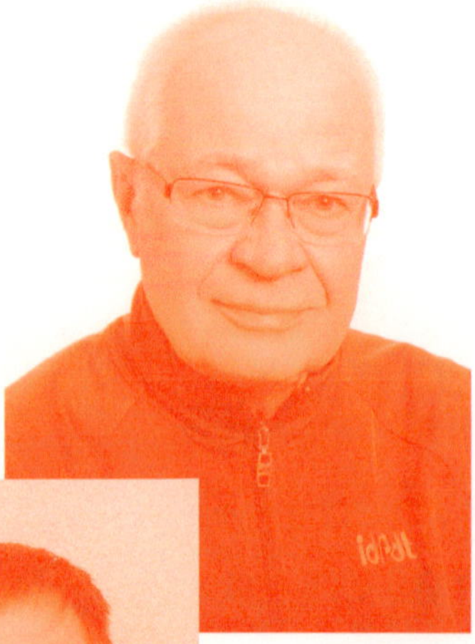
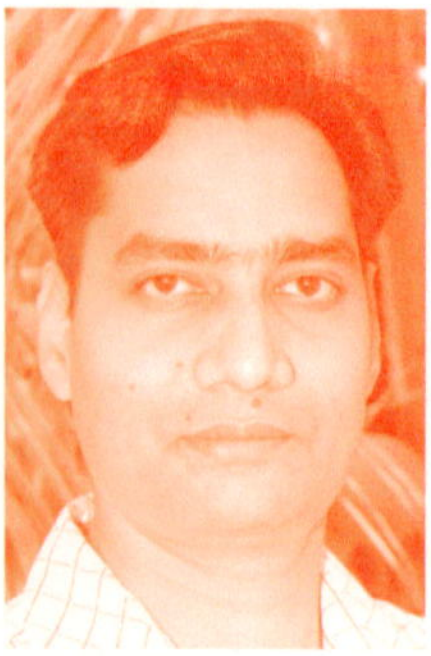
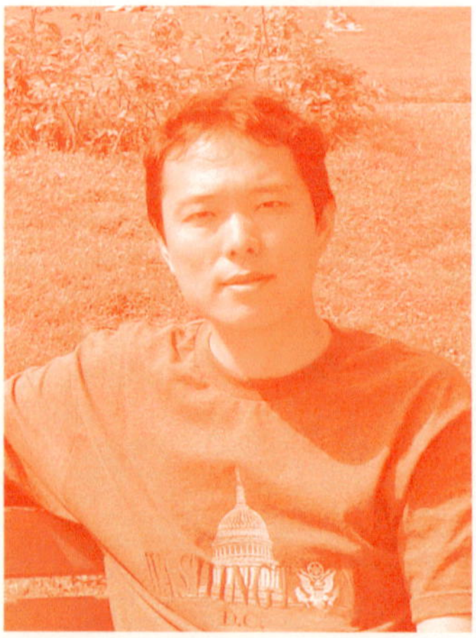
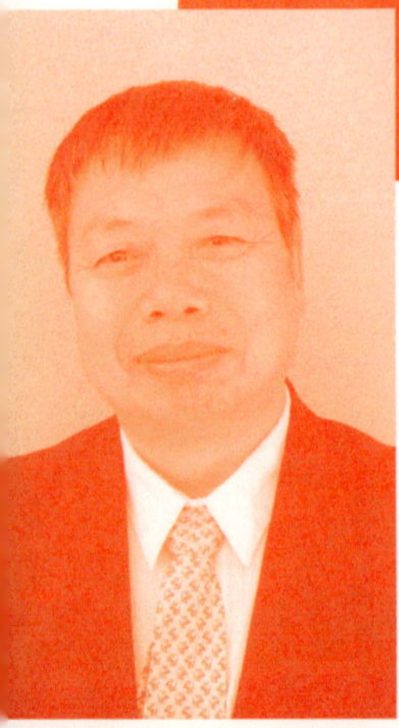
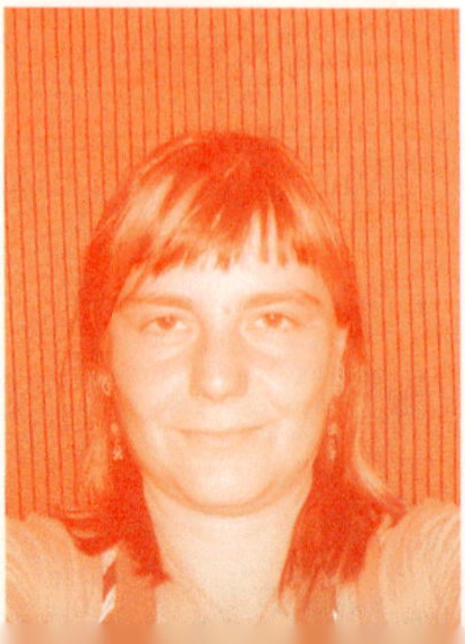

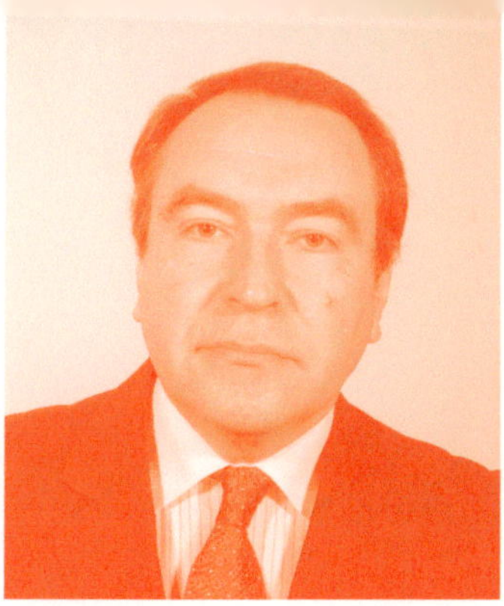
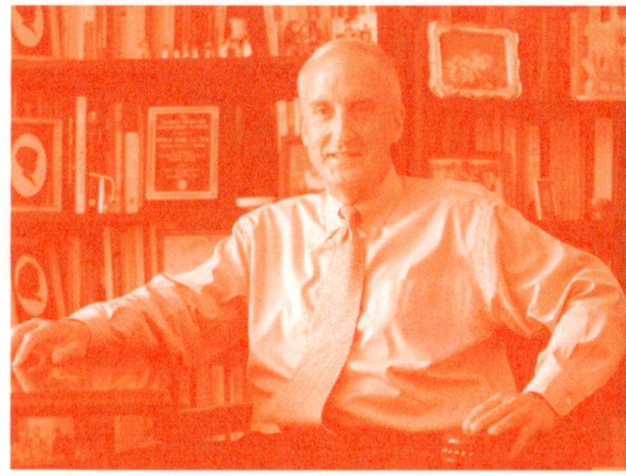
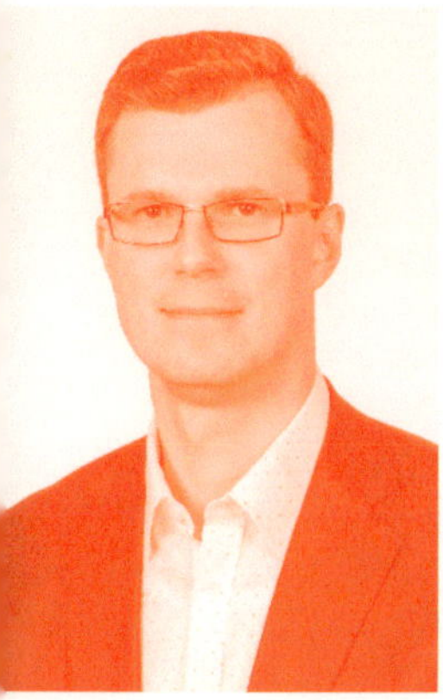
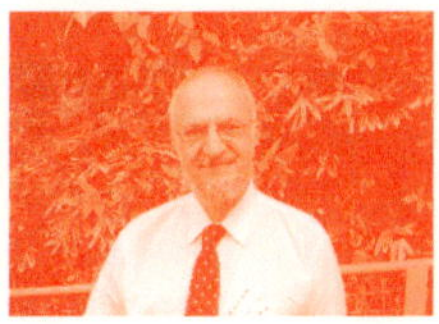
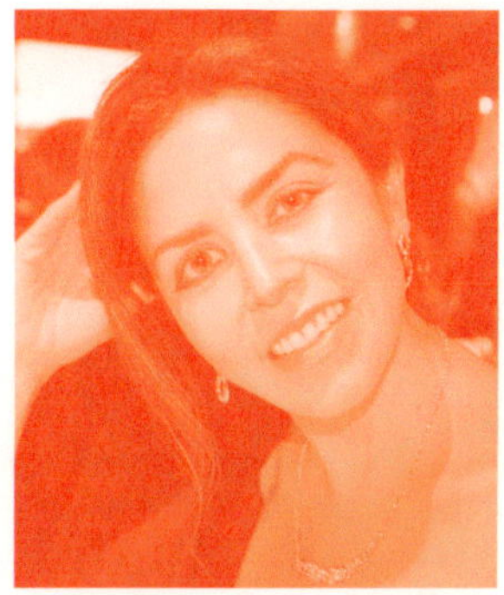

Supporting open minds since 2005

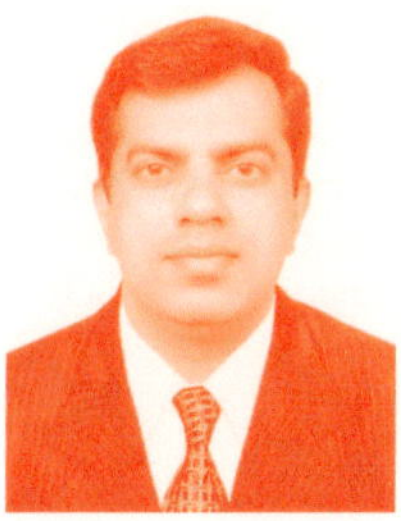
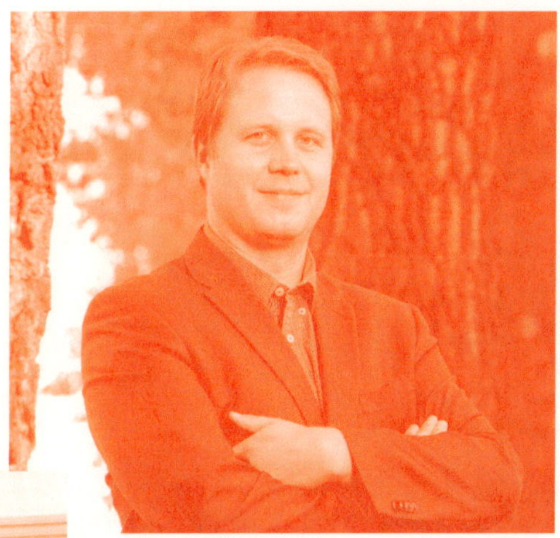
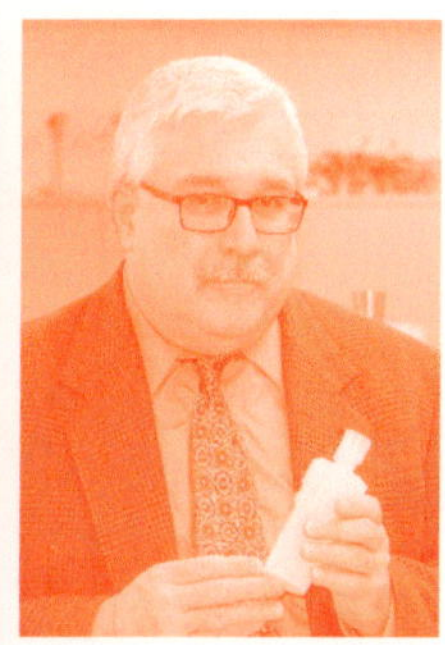
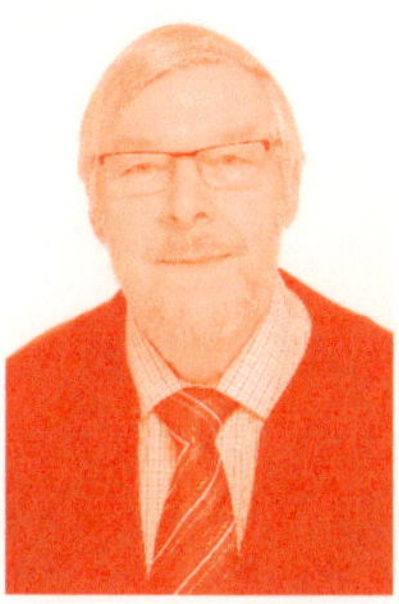
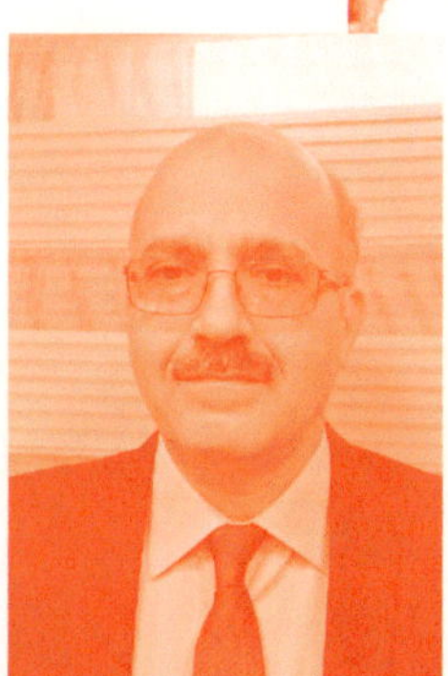
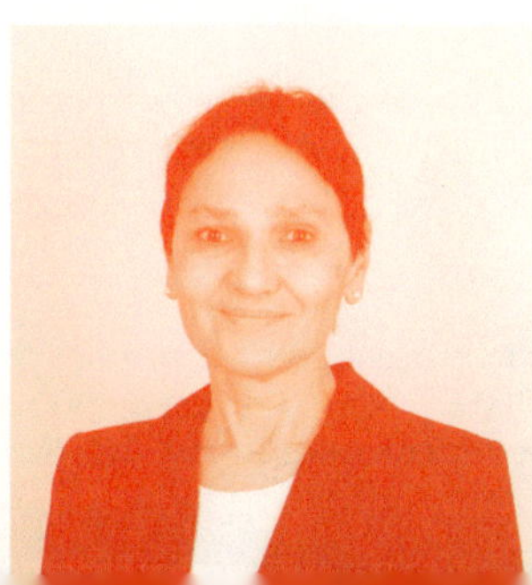
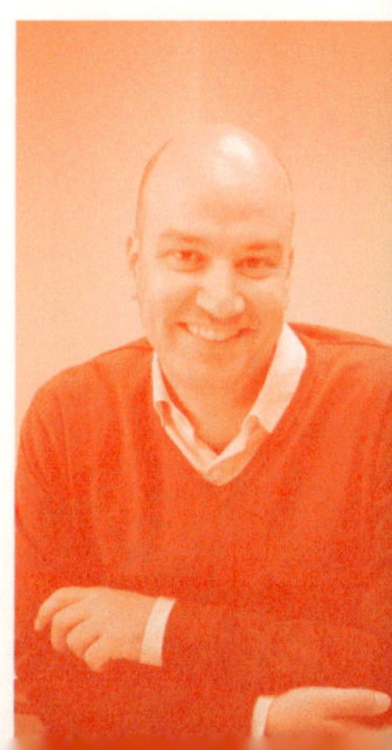

Cardiac Arrhythmias - Translational Approach from Pathophysiology to Advanced Care
http://dx.doi.org/10.5772/intechopen.94674
Edited by Endre Zima

Contributors
Dmytro Skoryi, Dmytro Volkov, Iurii Karpenko, Amad Hania, Bin Liu, Brian D. Tow, Ingrid M. Bonilla, Sombat Muengtaweepongsa, Dilok Piyayotai, Srinivasan Jayaraman, Ponnuraj Kirthi Priya, Zuraini Md. Noor, Raj Parikh, Meher Singha, Abhishek Madathanapalli, Endre Zima, Bettina Nagy, Boldizsár Kiss, Gábor Áron Fülöp

First published in London, United Kingdom, 2022 by IntechOpen
IntechOpen is the global imprint of INTECHOPEN LIMITED, registered in England and Wales, registration number: 11086078, 5 Princes Gate Court, London, SW7 2QJ, United Kingdom
Printed in Croatia

British Library Cataloguing-in-Publication Data
A catalogue record for this book is available from the British Library

Additional hard and PDF copies can be obtained from orders@intechopen.com

Cardiac Arrhythmias - Translational Approach from Pathophysiology to Advanced Care
Edited by Endre Zima
p. cm.
Print ISBN 978-1-83969-505-6
Online ISBN 978-1-83969-506-3
eBook (PDF) ISBN 978-1-83969-507-0

For EU product safety concerns:
IN TECH d.o.o., Prolaz Marije Krucifikse Kozulić 3, 51000 Rijeka, Croatia, info@intechopen.com or visit our website at intechopen.com.

Meet the editor

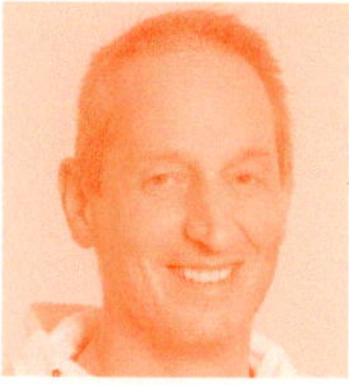

Endre Zima, MD, is head of Cardiac ICU at Semmelweis University Heart and Vascular Center, Budapest, Hungary. He is specialized in anesthesiology, intensive care, and cardiology. He received a Ph.D. in 2006 and a medical habilitation degree in 2017 from Semmelweis University. As a professor, he has been holding graduate and postgraduate lectures and practices in anesthesiology/intensive care and cardiology. He has a European Heart Rhythm Association (EHRA) accreditation for Cardiac Pacing and Implantable Cardioverter Defibrillators and is a Full Instructor of Advanced Life Support (ALS) and Basic Life Support (BLS) for the European Resuscitation Council. Dr. Zima is a fellow of the European Society of Cardiology, EHRA, and the Acute Cardiovascular Care Association. He is also the president of the Working Group on Cardiac Arrhythmias and Pacing and a board member of the Hungarian Society of Cardiology and WG of Heart Failure. His fields of research are acute and intensive cardiac care, cardiogenic shock/acute heart failure, cardiopulmonary resuscitation, post-cardiac arrest intensive care, invasive hemodynamic monitoring, arrhythmias, ICD/IPG/CRT therapy, and defibrillator waveform development. Dr. Zima has one accepted and one submitted patents patent to his credit. He is the author of thirteen book chapters, sixty-six international journal articles, and fifty-six native-language papers. He is currently supervising the research works of three Ph.D. students and seven medical students.

Contents

Preface

Knowledge of cardiac arrhythmias has significantly improved in the last several decades. Although most cases are benign and easy to evaluate and treat, arrhythmias are sometimes challenging to differentiate, requiring quick recognition and response. The worst-case scenario is a hemodynamically unstable arrhythmia that may lead to heart failure or cardiac arrest that necessitates cardiopulmonary resuscitation and complex intensive care.

A translational approach means implementing laboratory science into real-life clinical practice. Improvements in the science of arrhythmias have led to a decrease in morbidity and even mortality. Efforts to understand arrhythmic mechanisms have led to experimental modelling of arrhythmogenesis. These models are based on hypoxic-ischemic reperfusion myocardial insult, arrhythmogenic stimulating factors induced by electrolyte imbalance or administration of certain drugs. Over the last fifteen years, new methods of genetic testing have been developed that reveal new hereditary factors behind arrhythmias (e.g., cardiomyopathies), though genetics-driven therapy is still lacking.

The key to the effective and appropriate treatment of clinical arrhythmias is the identification of etiology. The classical diagnosis is based on a thorough analysis of the patient's ECG. Causative therapy is driven by further clinical examination, laboratory testing of blood samples, imaging studies (e.g., echocardiography, CT and MRI scans), and invasive cardiac procedures. Patients suffering from arrhythmic cardiac arrest require immediate diagnostics and therapeutics regardless of setting in order to increase their chances of survival.

This book contains eight chapters in which the contributing authors highlight special aspects of the current scientific knowledge on cardiac arrhythmias.

The molecular background of catecholaminergic and calcium-dependent ventricular tachycardias is a point of interest since the latter may lead to sudden cardiac death. Genetic mutations in components of the calcium signaling pathway may induce dysregulation of calcium leading to overload, and this may be the pathway to target for therapy. Ryanodine receptors could be useful interventional gates to prevent catecholaminergic ventricular arrhythmias.

The COVID-19 pandemic has devastated daily medical and social life. Affecting mainly the respiratory tract and causing acute respiratory distress syndrome (ARDS), COVID infection has direct and indirect effects on the heart itself via secondary thrombogenicity, ischemia, myocarditis, and electrical inhomogeneity. The newly developed antiviral agents have potential proarrhythmic effects with or without the ischemic insult of the myocardial tissue. This proarrhythmic burden spurred scientists to begin using an endo-, mid myo-, and epicardial myocyte anisotropic preparation model for testing the safety of the first-used "anti-COVID" agent hydroxychloroquine. The latter acts electrophysiologically differently on myocardial cells in hypokalemic, COVID-associated ischemic, or overdosed circumstances.

Bradycardia and heart failure together may be treated by cardiac implantable electronic devices (CIEDs). The pacing provides a better hemodynamic response, which is the aim of treating heart failure when the near-physiologic pacing sites are selected. To date, the first choice of device therapy for heart failure and the wide QRS complex is cardiac resynchronization therapy. "New-old" pacing methods are also tested to achieve better cardiac performance. The concept of pacing the bundle of His or left bundle branch has had a renaissance in the last five years. Despite the obvious benefits of pacing through the natural pacing conduction system of the heart, there are controversies on the skill-based and technical possibilities of it, limiting the widespread usage of the method.

Many supraventricular tachycardic arrhythmias have anatomical foci or accessory pathways in the background proven by electrophysiological diagnostic procedures. Most of these e.g. atrioventricular nodal reentrant tachycardia, atrioventricular reentrant tachycardia, atrial flutter, and atrial fibrillation can be treated by radiofrequency ablation. Few types of ventricular arrhythmias are also candidates for radiofrequency ablation, but most of them are treated with an implantable cardioverter-defibrillator (ICD) in addition to antiarrhythmic drug treatment. ICD was developed for primary and secondary prevention of ventricular arrhythmias and sudden cardiac death (SCD).

Sudden cardiac arrest is a major cause of mortality in developed countries. The incidence of out-of-hospital cardiac arrest is between 60 and 170 per 100,000 persons worldwide. Since the medical team is not present at the time of circulatory collapse in most cases, survival depends on the awareness and training of the people around the patient when the arrest occurs. Therefore, it is important to emphasize the relevance of the knowledge of the non-medical public recognizing cardiac arrest and providing basic life support until the emergency medical team arrives. The program of public access to automated defibrillators has also improved SCD mortality. In the era of widespread media coverage, more focus has been placed on SCD among athletes. Extreme sports activity, increased adrenaline release, lactic acidosis, and volume-electrolyte shifts may trigger SCD, which may be the first sign of undiagnosed heart disease in apparently healthy athletes. New guidelines in sports medicine suggest thorough examination and screening for underlying asymptomatic cardiac disorders.

Arrhythmias may cause a peri-arrest state or cardiac arrest in the hospital, intensive care unit, or even during anesthesia. Most of these cases occur because of stress due to surgery or hemostasis, volume, and electrolyte disorders, which are to be treated or corrected during the treatment of malignant arrhythmias.

After successful resuscitation, when the patient has returned the spontaneous circulation (ROSC), a special global systemic-ischemic reperfusion syndrome-induced multiple organ dysfunction may develop, which is defined as post-cardiac arrest syndrome. All the causative reversible factors should be promptly recognized and corrected to avoid the relapse of circulatory arrest. To prevent ischemic-reperfusion brain injury, a neuroprotective target temperature management (formerly mild therapeutic hypothermia) is part of the intensive care of patients suffering from a long-standing no-flow or low-flow perfusion before ROSC. These patients need special post-resuscitation intensive care, sedation, mechanical ventilation, and temperature management. As such, prognosis is difficult to estimate during the first 72–120 hours. Special protocols for prognostication cover the clinical neurological judgment, EEG, imaging modalities, and special neuron-specific biomarkers.

In conclusion, the translational approach to cardiac arrhythmias highlights interesting aspects of arrhythmia mechanisms as well as diagnostic and therapeutic methods. This book emphasizes a quick, critical, and thorough response to arrhythmias to prevent further deterioration of the patient. Knowledge of the basic molecular, cellular, and clinical background of arrhythmias is the foundation of clinical appraisal and treatment.

Endre Zima MD, Ph.D., Dr. med. habil.
Professor,
Consultant Anesthesiologist,
Intensive Care Specialist and Cardiologist,
Head of Cardiac Intensive Care Unit,
Heart and Vascular Center,
Semmelweis University,
Budapest, Hungary

Chapter 1

Molecular Mechanism and Current Therapies for Catecholaminergic Polymorphic Ventricular Tachycardia

Bin Liu, Brian D. Tow and Ingrid M. Bonilla

Abstract

The rhythmic contraction of the heart relies on tightly regulated calcium (Ca) release from the sarcoplasmic reticulum (SR) Ca release channel, Ryanodine receptor (RyR2). Genetic mutations in components of the calcium release unit such as RyR2, cardiac calsequestrin and other proteins have been shown to cause a genetic arrhythmic syndrome known as catecholaminergic polymorphic ventricular tachycardia (CPVT). This book chapter will focus on the following: (1) to describing CPVT as a stress-induced cardiac arrhythmia syndrome and its genetic causes. (2) Discussing the regulation of SR Ca release, and how dysregulation of Ca release contributes to arrhythmogenesis. (3) Discussing molecular mechanisms of CPVT with a focus on impaired Ca signaling refractoriness as a unifying mechanism underlying different genetic forms of CPVT. (4) Discussing pharmacological approaches as CPVT treatments as well as other potential future therapies. Since dysregulated SR Ca release has been implicated in multiple cardiac disorders including heart failure and metabolic heart diseases, knowledge obtained from CPVT studies will also shed light on the development of therapeutic approaches for these devastating cardiac dysfunctions as a whole.

Keywords: EC coupling, Ca-dependent arrhythmias, RyR2, Ca signaling, sudden cardiac death, DCR

1. Introduction

The rhythmic beating of the heart is controlled by an intricate and well-orchestrated flux of ions through a process called excitation–contraction coupling (ECC), where the electrical action potential leads to cellular contraction. Among all the ions involved in ECC, calcium (Ca) plays a critical role and serves as the signal for cardiac contraction. Briefly, upon cardiac excitation a small current of Ca enters the cytoplasm through the sarcolemmal L-type Ca channels (LTCC). This triggers a much larger Ca release from the sarcoplasmic reticulum (SR)—the intracellular Ca store—by opening the type 2 ryanodine receptor (RyR2) channel in a process called Ca-induced-Ca release (CICR) [1]. The resultant elevation of cytoplasmic Ca concentration activates the contractile apparatus, thus leading to myocyte contraction. For relaxation to occur, Ca must be extruded from the cytoplasm. Two main

 IntechOpen

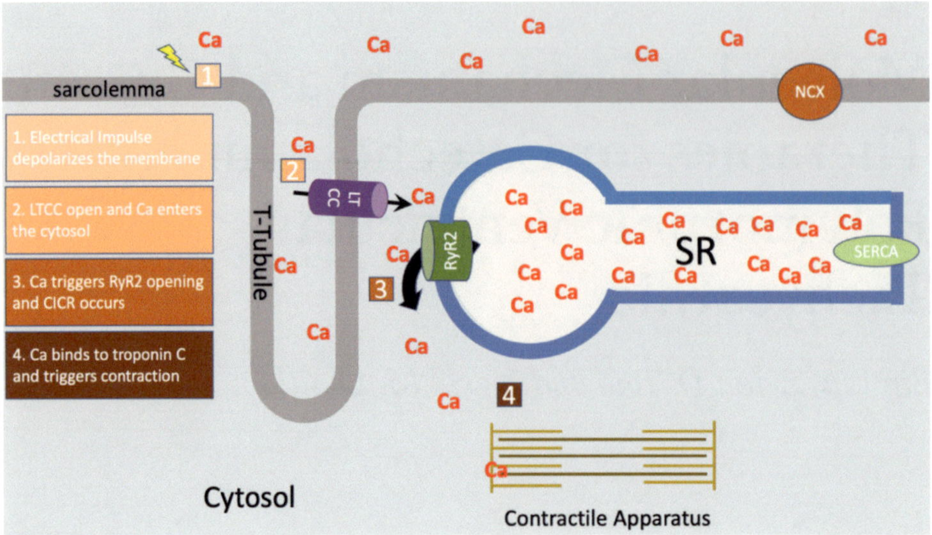

Figure 1.
Cardiac excitation-contraction coupling.

mechanisms are involved in removing cytoplasmic Ca: one is by Ca re-sequestration into the SR to replenish the intracellular store, through the action of the SR Ca ATPase (SERCA). The other is by transporting calcium outside of the cell via the membrane-embedded protein, sodium calcium exchanger (NCX) (**Figure 1**). Other avenues for Ca removal do exist (e.g. sarcolemmal Ca-ATPase and mitochondria Ca uniporter), but only play a minor role in this process [1]. The rhythmic rise and fall of cytoplasmic Ca underlies the systolic and diastolic phases of the cardiac cycle.

2. Dysregulated SR Ca release is linked to cardiac pathologies

The RyR2 is a large protein with a molecular weight of ~560 kDa that forms homotetrameric channels in the SR membrane (**Figure 2**) [2]. Due to its crucial role in releasing Ca to trigger contraction, it is no surprise that there are a number of auxiliary proteins with likely overlapping/redundant functions acting from both the cytosolic and SR luminal sides to regulate the function of the channel complex. Moreover, the activity of the channel is also subject to regulation by post-translational modifications, including redox modifications, phosphorylation, and nitrosylation [3]. Unfortunately, both genetic and acquired defects due to mutation or posttranslational modification of the channel complex contribute to its dysfunction [3]. These defects typically make the channel hyperactive or leaky, giving rise to dysregulated Ca release (DCR). DCR is implicated in a spectrum of cardiac dysfunctions [3], and in particular, it directly causes a deadly cardiac arrhythmia syndrome, catecholaminergic polymorphic ventricular tachycardia (CPVT) [3, 4].

CPVT is a stress-induced arrhythmia that is triggered by elevated levels of catecholamines [5]. Patients do not exhibit the cardiac remodeling typical of structural heart diseases, which makes the diagnosis particularly challenging. Life-threatening cardiac arrhythmias occur following exercise or emotional stress, which elevates circulating catecholamine levels. CPVT mutations have been identified in the genes encoding the RyR2 channel and its several auxiliary proteins. The remainder of this chapter focuses on the regulation of SR Ca release, the molecular mechanisms of CPVT, and the current and future state of therapies targeted towards CPVT.

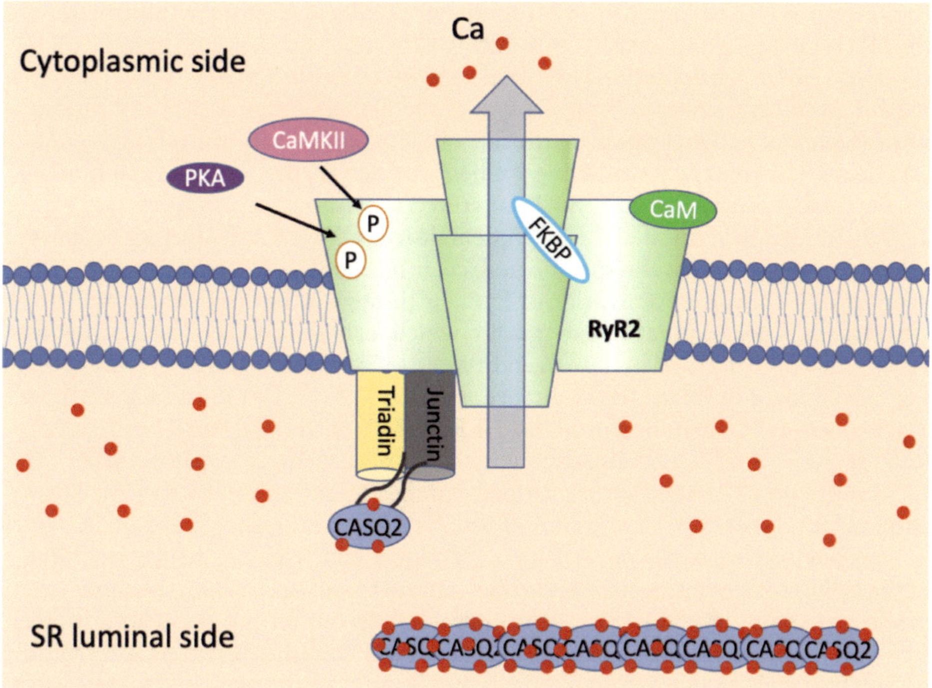

Figure 2.
SR Ca release channel RyR2 is regulated by both cytosolic and SR luminal proteins.

Since dysregulated SR Ca release has been implicated in multiple cardiac disorders, knowledge obtained from CPVT studies will also shed light on the development of therapeutic approaches for these devastating cardiac dysfunctions as a whole.

3. Modulation of RyR2 Ca release

RyR2s form physically separated/isolated clusters to act as functionally independent Ca release units [6]. Within dyads, the structural element formed by the close apposition of T-tubules and junctional SR, Ca influx via LTCC in the T-tubule triggers more Ca release from RyR2 clusters in the junctional SR to initiate contraction (**Figure 1**). Ca release from individually activated RyR2 clusters are known as Ca sparks and can be experimentally observed during diastole [7]. The systolic Ca transient is the summation of tens of thousands of Ca sparks due to the synchronized Ca release of RyR2 clusters following sarcolemmal depolarization. The positive-feedback nature of CICR suggests that SR Ca release should terminate upon depletion of SR Ca store. However, only a fraction of the SR Ca store is released during EC coupling [8, 9]. This begs the question of how the Ca release process is terminated. Cytosolic Ca-dependent inactivation of RyR2 has been proposed as a mechanism for the termination of Ca release [10], but lacks widespread support. In contrast, evidence from different research groups collectively points to a mechanism that works to inhibit Ca release from the SR luminal side.

The first piece of evidence comes from an *in vitro* study conducted with single RyR2 channels reconstituted into lipid bilayers. This study demonstrated that the opening of RyR2 is significantly reduced at lowered luminal Ca [11]. The channel's luminal accessory proteins, calsequestrin 2 (CASQ2), junctin, and triadin, are required for this luminal Ca-dependent inhibition of the channel [12]. More convincing evidence comes from a subsequent cellular study that manipulated the SR Ca buffering capacity by introducing exogenous Ca chelators into the SR to result in a slower Ca depletion [13]. Enhanced SR Ca buffering drastically increased the amplitude of Ca release (both Ca sparks and global Ca transients) and slowed its termination, hence supporting the role of SR luminal Ca in controlling RyR2 Ca release. Mathematical modelling studies provided further support that luminal Ca-dependent deactivation of RyR2 is involved in termination of Ca release [14].

While the role of luminal Ca-dependent deactivation of RyR2 has been established, it is unclear what the specific molecular mechanism is. There is evidence supporting either direct activation of RyR2 or through its luminal accessory proteins, i.e. CASQ2, junctin, and triadin, which form the SR Ca release unit with RyR2. Studies performed in human embryonic kidney cells (HEK293) overexpressing recombinant RyR2 support a direct activation of RyR2 by luminal Ca. Despite a lack of several Ca handling proteins, HEK293 cells with exogenously expressed RyR2 mutants of CPVT exhibit dysregulated Ca release that is sensitive to SR Ca load in a process called store-overload-induced Ca release (SOICR) [15]. The authors found that CPVT mutations of RyR2 reduce the threshold for SOICR, which is expected to increase the propensity of dysregulated Ca release, hence contributing to cellular arrhythmogenesis. Further, a more recent study from the same group proposed the amino acid E4872 as the luminal Ca sensor for the direct activation of RyR2 [16]. A point mutation of E4872A completely abolishes luminal Ca activation of RyR2 in single channel studies, and markedly reduces dysregulated Ca release in HEK293 and HL-1 cardiac cells. Moreover, mice harboring a heterozygous mutation of E4872Q are resistant to SOICR and protected from ventricular arrhythmias *in vivo*. E4872 is localized in the S6 helix bundle-crossing region, the putative cation binding pocket of RyR2. Despite recent breakthroughs in resolving the structure of RyR2, the composition of this putative cation binding pocket remains undetermined [17], and it is thought that other key amino acids in this region such as E4878 may also play a critical role in luminal Ca activation of RyR2.

On the other hand, independent labs have provided evidence supporting the participation of luminal proteins in regulating RyR2 Ca release. Lipid bilayer single-channel studies found that CASQ2 serves as a sensor to inhibit opening of RyR2 at low luminal [Ca], which notably required the presence of junctin and triadin, thus suggesting these proteins form a regulatory complex to control luminal Ca-dependent deactivation of RyR2 [12]. Additionally, increasing or decreasing the expression of CASQ2 in rat cardiac myocyte not only changes the SR Ca storage capacity, consistent with CASQ2's Ca buffer function, but also affects SR Ca release [18]. In particular, decreased expression of CASQ2 leads to dysregulated arrhythmogenic Ca release, supporting CASQ2 function as an inhibitor of RyR2 [18]. Interestingly, the expression of a competitive peptide in myocytes to disrupt the interaction between CASQ2 and triadin impairs the ability of CASQ2 to stabilize the Ca release channel [19], thus echoing conclusions from earlier bilayer studies that CASQ2 interacts with other luminal proteins to regulate RyR2 activity. The development of a genetic model of CASQ2 KO mouse provided additional evidence supporting CASQ2's regulation of SR Ca release [20]. CASQ2 KO mice phenocopied human CPVT by exhibiting catecholamine-induced tachyarrhythmias in vivo. Myocytes isolated from these mice are characterized with β agonist-induced dysregulated Ca release, a hallmark of cellular arrhythmogenesis. However, besides resulting in CPVT, the ablation of major SR Ca buffer protein CASQ2 does not seem to result in more severe cardiac dysfunctions, suggesting the existence of other Ca buffer proteins with similar function at the SR luminal side. Surprisingly, deletion of CASQ2 and another Ca binding protein histidine-rich calcium binding protein (HRC) in a double knockout (DKO) mouse model alleviates arrhythmias as compared with the CASQ2 KO mouse [21]. HRC binds to RyR2 through the same CASQ2-binding domain on triadin, and results from this DKO mouse study suggest that rather than having redundant roles, CASQ2 and HRC play opposing roles to regulate RyR2 Ca release. Taken together, these studies not only support the notion that luminal accessory proteins of RyR2 participate in controlling SR Ca release, but also highlight the intricate nature of such regulation.

4. Molecular mechanisms of CPVT

CPVT mutations have been identified in 6 genes encoding 4 different proteins of the Ca release channel complex: *RYR2*, *CASQ2*, *TRDN*, *CALM1*, *CALM2*, and *CALM3* [22]. Among them, the 3 genes of calmodulin (*CALM1*, *CALM2*, and *CALM3*) encode the same protein. Of note, these mutations account for up to 60–75% of CPVT cases, with the genetic cause of the remaining clinical cases unknown [23, 24]. It is likely that more disease mutations will be discovered in other proteins of the Ca release channel complex. In this section, we will summarize the proposed molecular mechanisms for different genetic forms of CPVT.

4.1 CPVT linked to RyR2 mutations

Among the genetically confirmed cases of CPVT, over 90% are due to mutations of RyR2 [23]. CPVT linked to RyR2 mutations is autosomal dominant. Up to date, more than 200 gain-of-function mutations in RyR2 have been discovered. RyR2 loss-of-function mutations have also been detected but are less frequent and are associated with arrhythmias distinct from CPVT [25]. Additionally, the loss-of-function mutation appears to cause arrhythmias through an early afterdepolarization (EAD)-based mechanism [26] which is much less studied compared to the classic DAD-based mechanism. Never the less, EADs have been observed in CPVT patient specific induced pluripotent stem cells (iPSC)-derived cardiomyocytes [27] in addition to myocytes isolated from a mouse model harboring a loss-of-function CPVT mutation of RyR2 [26]. The focus of the rest of the chapter will be on the arrhythmias evoked by DADs, rather than EADs.

Three main theories of how gain-of-function RyR2 mutations lead to CPVT have been proposed by different groups. The first comes from the observation that CPVT mutants of RyR2 expressed in HEK293 cells decreased the threshold to induce SOICR [15]. Based on these results, it is proposed that CPVT mutations make RyR2 more sensitive to luminal Ca, thus susceptible to dysregulated arrhythmogenic Ca release. The second theory proposes that CPVT mutations reduce the binding of RyR2 to FKBP12.6, a cytosolic protein thought to stabilize the channel, thus increasing RyR2 activity and giving rise to arrhythmogenic diastolic calcium release [28]. However, this theory has been challenged by several labs [29–31], a conserved binding between CPVT mutant RyR2 and FKBP has been reported [32]. The majority of RyR2 mutations are found at three "hot spots" which are located in the N-terminal domain (amino acids 1–600), central domain (amino acids ~2100–2500) and C terminal domain (amino acids ~3900–end) of the protein [33, 34]. Structural studies show that many of them are found at the domain-domain interfaces, thus giving rise to the third theory that mutations impair the inter-domain interactions of RyR2 to cause CPVT. Specifically, the interaction between N-terminal and central domains of RyR2 is responsible for the so-called domain "zipping" and is thought to stabilize the channel; the third theory posits that CPVT mutants impair this interaction (causing domain unzipping) and causes channel dysfunction. This model of domain zipping-unzipping has been supported by experimental evidence [35–37].

4.2 CPVT linked to CASQ2 mutations

The second most common cause of CPVT is mutation of CASQ2, an SR luminal Ca binding protein thought to regulate deactivation of RyR2. CPVT linked to CASQ2 was considered as an autosomal recessive disease until the recent discovery of autosomal dominant disease-causing mutations [38]. CASQ2 is a low-affinity, high-capacity Ca binding protein. It does not contain Ca binding structural domains such as an EF-hand motif, a helix–loop–helix structural domain, found in "typical" Ca binding proteins (troponin C, calmodulin) [39]. Instead, it has multiple (~60–70) negatively charged amino acids, which facilitates electrostatic interactions between the protein and ~ 40–50 Ca ions [40]. CASQ2 monomers change their structure upon Ca binding, and form protein polymers in a Ca-dependent process. Structural studies show that monomeric CASQ2 contains three highly similar tandem domains, resembling that of bacterial thioredoxin. However, much less is known about the structure of the polymers. Based on *in vitro* biophysical studies by Park et al. [41], the following model of CASQ2 polymerization is proposed: CASQ2s exist as monomers at low luminal [Ca]; as [Ca] increases, CASQ2s form dimers, tetramers, and polymers in a [Ca]-dependent process. Thus, CASQ2s polymerize to bind additional Ca at high luminal Ca, but depolymerize to release Ca at low luminal Ca. Considering the Ca and protein concentrations in SR, CASQ2s likely exist as a mixture of monomers, dimers, and polymers of varying sizes [42]. As described above, monomeric CASQ2 is thought to be anchored to RyR2 via junctin and triadin to deactivate Ca release at low luminal Ca. The intriguing question remains whether this Ca-dependent change in the polymerization states of CASQ2 happens on a beat-to-beat basis in response to SR Ca load to regulate RyR2 Ca release. It has been shown that the polymerization state of CASQ2 changes upon depletion of luminal Ca in fibroblast by fluorescent approaches [43]. Additional evidence comes from studies conducted with skeletal muscle fibers demonstrating luminal-Ca dependent changes in polymerization of CASQ1, the skeletal counterpart of CASQ2 [44]. However, whether Ca-dependent changes in CASQ2 polymerization happens in beating cardiomyocytes at a time scale comparable with the cardiac cycle awaits further investigation.

At least 2 molecular mechanisms are proposed to explain how autosomal recessive CPVT mutations of CASQ2 cause the disease based on its two primary functions, buffering Ca and modulating RyR2 opening [4]. These mutations (nonsense or missense) lead to loss or reduced expression of CASQ2. Subsequently, reduced Ca buffering allows the free Ca to rise faster near the Ca release sites, thereby triggering dysregulated Ca release. Besides reduced Ca buffering power, some missense mutations of CASQ2 appear to work through another mechanism: by impairing RyR2 regulation from the luminal side. It's been shown that the mutation of R33Q leads to abnormal interaction between CASQ2 and the Ca release channel complex [45], and another mutation of D307H reduces the binding between CASQ2 and triadin [46]. These results support the notion that a regulatory complex involving several proteins (CASQ2, triadin, junctin, and potentially others) senses luminal Ca to regulate Ca release, and disruption of interactions between them leads to dysregulation of the channel and disease. Compared with the autosomal recessive mutations, less is known about the autosomal dominant mutations that were more recently identified. Two mutations (K180R and S173I) have been found to interfere the polymerization of CASQ2 [47], likely causing CPVT by reducing the Ca buffering capacity.

4.3 CPVT linked to triadin mutations

CPVT mutations have also been identified in triadin, a trans-SR membrane protein that helps anchor CASQ2 to the RyR2 channel complex. Triadin has a short

N-terminal region located on the cytosolic side of SR, a single membrane spanning domain, and a highly charged C-terminal region that comprises most of the protein and resides in the SR luminal side. The C-terminal tail of the protein contains KEKE motifs formed by stretches of alternating residues with opposite charges. A single KEKE motif consisting of 15 residues (210–224) has been suggested as the CASQ2 binding region [48]. The binding between triadin and CASQ2 is Ca-dependent and they dissociate at high [Ca] (10 mM). In contrast, triadin's binding to RyR2 is Ca-independent [48]. Due to its role of anchoring CASQ2 to Ca release sites, triadin is thought to facilitate SR Ca release by allowing CASQ2 to buffer Ca near the Ca release channel.

It is also proposed that triadin may play a direct role in regulating RyR2 channel activity. Both overexpression and knockout mouse models of triadin have been created to decipher its function. The overexpression model displayed hypertrophy and altered Ca handling, accompanied by compensatory changes in the expression of several proteins of the RyR2 channel complex, thus masking the functional role of triadin [49]. Similarly, loss of triadin in the KO model also caused compensatory changes [50]. Drastic reduction in the interface of junctional SR and T-tubules occurred due to structural remodeling, thus impaired the coupling between RyR2 and LTCC. As a result, inactivation of LTCC is reduced, which increased Ca current, prolonged action potential, and subsequently increased cellular and SR Ca. Due to Ca overload, myocytes from triadin KO model displayed elevated levels of arrhythmogenic Ca release, especially when stimulated with catecholamines [50]. While both mouse models support the notion that triadin plays an important role in myocyte Ca handling, the massive compensatory changes in these chronic models makes an explanation of the data challenging. Nevertheless, acute overexpression of triadin in cultured myocytes increased RyR2 opening, dysregulated Ca release, and membrane depolarization, mimicking the cellular phenotype of CPVT [51]. Relatively few CPVT mutations of triadin have been reported as of yet. In a 2012 study, three autosomal recessive mutations of triadin were discovered, with two of them (one deletion, one nonsense) resulting in loss of the protein. The third one, a missense mutation of T59R, results in a protein that is more susceptible to degradation [52]. Thus, loss or decreased expression of triadin appear to cause CPVT. Another two autosomal recessive triadin mutations were identified in a 2015 study [53], although the underlying disease-causing mechanisms await further investigation.

4.4 CPVT linked to calmodulin mutations

Calmodulin (CaM) is an EF-hand Ca binding protein that binds RyR2 from the cytosolic side to regulate Ca release. CaM has a dumbbell-shaped structure, with its two globular domains connected by a flexible central helix. Each of the two domains contain two EF-hand Ca binding sites. The N-domain of the protein has a lower Ca binding affinity than the C-domain [54, 55]. Upon Ca binding, the hydrophobic pockets in both domains become exposed, thereby allowing CaM to bind its several intracellular targets, including RyR2, LTCC and Na channel (Nav 1.5) [56]. Mutations of CaM have been linked to different types of arrhythmias, such as CPVT, long QT syndrome, and idiopathic ventricular fibrillation, likely due to its impaired regulation of various target proteins [22]. Following systolic Ca release and the ensuing increasing in Ca on the cytosolic side of RyR2, CaM binds to the channel and inhibits its opening during the diastole phase of the cardiac cycle [57, 58]. CPVT mutations of CaM appear to have impaired ability to inhibit the channel and promoted the generation of DCR in the form of Ca waves and Ca sparks in a cellular study [59]. They also exhibited higher binding affinity to RyR2 than WT CaM, thereby contributing to the autosomal dominant mode of action [59].

5. Impaired Ca signaling refractoriness and generation of DCR

Despite the differences in the molecular details on how the various CPVT mutations of the RyR2 channel complex cause the disease, they all seem to make the channel more susceptible to arrhythmogenic diastolic Ca release. Following systolic Ca release, RyR2 becomes functionally suppressed and remains that way for a brief period, known as Ca signaling refractoriness [60]. Refractoriness of the Ca release channel can be measured by myocyte experiments employing a two-pulse protocol to record the process of Ca transient restitution. It's been demonstrated that full recovery of Ca transient takes ~1 s (anywhere from ~0.8 – 1.5 s, depending on species) [61–65]. If Ca signaling refractoriness is impaired, the RyR2 channel is expected to recover earlier from the functionally suppressed state, thereby promoting the generation of DCR, thus causing cellular arrhythmogenesis. Indeed, multiple CPVT mutations have been found to shorten refractoriness of RyR2, including mutations of CASQ2 [65], CaM [66], and RyR2 [67]. Moreover, shortened Ca signaling refractoriness can also occur due to oxidation/hyperphosphorylation of RyR2 as seen in models of acquired heart diseases [63]. Thus, both genetic and acquired defects of RyR2 channel complex seem to converge on shortening Ca signaling refractoriness to cause arrhythmogenic Ca release. Further evidence supporting shortened refractoriness as a unifying mechanism for the generation of DCR comes from a recent study using an engineered therapeutic CaM in an attempt to restore refractoriness and treat CPVT [66], as discussed in a later section on future therapies for CPVT. Taken together, these studies suggest that disease mutations may change the SR Ca dynamics, the modulation of RyR2 by cytosolic or luminal proteins, or conformational changes of the channel protein itself, each of which has been experimentally demonstrated to shorten Ca signaling refractoriness and give rise to arrhythmogenic DCR.

6. Cellular arrhythmogenesis: SR Ca load

At the single myocyte level, DCR is manifested as different forms: Ca sparks, Ca wavelets, and propagating Ca waves. When large enough, DCR activates electrogenic NCX, resulting in an inward current that causes delayed afterdepolarization (DAD) [68–70]. With a large enough amplitude, DADs may surpass the voltage threshold to open Na channels, thus leading to the generation of an ectopic action potential or triggered activity [71, 72]. Both the amplitude and the rate of DCRs are important in determining if it will trigger an ectopic action potential [73]. Localized DCR events in the form of Ca sparks and wavelets are less likely to trigger ectopic action potentials as compared with propagating Ca waves. Ca waves are more likely to occur when SR Ca load is high, such as following activation of β-adrenergic signaling pathways.

β-adrenergic stimulation results in phosphorylation of key EC-coupling proteins and subsequent generation of a larger and faster Ca transient, underlying its positive inotropy (ability to contract) and lusitropy (ability to relax) effect [1]. One of these proteins, phospholamban (PLN), acts as an inhibitor of SERCA. Its inhibition on SERCA is relieved upon β-adrenergic-dependent phosphorylation, thus contributing to a faster Ca transient decay and also higher SR Ca content. This higher SR Ca load facilitates Ca wave generation, and explains the stress-induced arrhythmias that occur in CPVT. Therefore, SERCA's function to refill the SR with Ca is critical to maintain a certain SR Ca load to stimulate the generation of Ca waves. On the other hand, SERCA directs Ca out of the cytosol while refilling the SR with Ca, which opposes the formation of or "breaks" Ca waves.

Based on these seemingly contradictory effects of SERCA activity on Ca wave generation, an interesting question arises: what will be the consequences of upregulating SERCA activity in the setting of CPVT? Both beneficial and deleterious effects have been reported from studies conducted by different groups. When overexpressing a skeletal isoform of SERCA1a in the CPVT model of CASQ2 KO, the resultant CPVT-SERCA^{ox} mice developed severe Ca-dependent cardiomyopathy [74]. These mice suffered from early mortality and contractile dysfunction. Myocytes isolated from the hypertrophied hearts of these animals also displayed enhanced levels of DCR. While these results clearly demonstrate a detrimental effect, the severe cardiomyopathy phenotype due to chronic SERCA overexpression masks the effect of the genetic manipulation on arrhythmias. A follow-up study from the same group conditionally overexpressed SERCA2a in the same CASQ2 KO mice and found that both atrial and ventricular arrhythmias were exacerbated due to acute upregulation of SERCA activity [75]. In contrast, in another study employing a different CPVT model of RyR2 knock in mouse (R4496C$^{+/-}$), upregulation of SERCA activity by knocking out its inhibitor PLN suppressed arrhythmias *in vivo*. In cellular experiments, Ca waves were also suppressed, due to propagating Ca waves being converted into non-arrhythmogenic mini waves and Ca sparks [76]. Interestingly, a different study showed that although enhancing SERCA activity by PLB ablation alleviated arrhythmias, it exacerbated myocardial infarction and cardiac damage in a RyR2 model featuring elevated DCR due to a mutation (S2814D) mimicking constitutive CaMKII-mediated phosphorylation of RyR2 [77].

7. Synchronization of DCR in myocardium

It is well established how DCR triggers ectopic action potentials at the cellular level. However, the heart contains billions of cardiomyocytes, and how arrhythmogenesis at the level of isolated myocytes translates into arrhythmias at the level of a multi-cellular tissue preparation or even the whole heart remains unknown. Within the myocardium, individual myocytes are electrically coupled to their neighboring cells, hence Ca-dependent depolarizing currents generated in any random, isolated cells should be easily absorbed by neighboring cells that act as a current sink (the source-sink mismatch theory) [78]. Therefore, cellular depolarization, if happening randomly in individual cells, cannot generate sufficient current to trigger tissue-level depolarization.

Computational simulation studies suggest a very large number of cells—nearly $7x10^5$—have to depolarize simultaneously to overcome source-sink mismatch and trigger depolarization to generate an ectopic beat in normal myocardium. This number is reduced by modeling disease conditions such as fibrosis or heart failure related electrical remodeling, but the number of requisite cells still remains quite large [78]. Therefore, it's been proposed that DCR happens in a synchronous way in multiple cells of the CPVT hearts to cause a tissue-wide ectopic beat. Experimental evidence has been provided in support of the synchronization of DCR in a CPVT model carrying the CASQ2 R33Q mutation [65]. This study quantified the degree of DCR synchronization by measuring the latency, or the time interval to the first DCR, following systolic Ca release. It was found that DCR occurs in a highly synchronized way in both myocytes and cardiac muscle tissue obtained from the R33Q CPVT model. Importantly, two factors are important for the synchronization of DCR: 1) shortened Ca signaling refractoriness that increases the propensity of release sites to fire synchronously by facilitating CICR, and 2) the presence of a preceding systolic action potential acting as a synchronizing event that temporally aligns the release sites and primes them for recovery from refractoriness.

8. The cellular origin of CPVT: Purkinje cells or ventricular myocytes?

Purkinje fibers are a specialized network of electrically excitable cells found in the conduction system of the heart. They radiate throughout the ventricular muscle to ensure a rapid propagation of electrical impulse and a coordinated ventricular contraction. Compared with the myocardium, the Purkinje system has a smaller source-sink mismatch [78]. Based on this and other structural features [79], Purkinje cells have been proposed as the cellular origin of many arrhythmias including CPVT. Experimental evidence obtained from the CPVT model of RyR2 R4496C$^{+/-}$ mouse supports this hypothesis [80]. Optical mapping of R4496C$^{+/-}$ hearts demonstrates that ventricular tachycardia (VT) may originate from the His-Purkinje system in both ventricles. Cellular studies also found that Purkinje cells had a significantly higher rate of DCR and triggered activity compared to ventricular myocytes [81, 82].

However, a recent study attempting to establish the causal link between Purkinje cells and CPVT did not provide such evidence [83]. In this study, CASQ2 was conditionally knocked out in the cardiac conduction system, but not the myocardium, using a conduction system-specific Cre recombinase. Ablation of CASQ2 in the Purkinje fibers failed to produce a CPVT phenotype. Considering CASQ2 ablation is an established molecular cause of CPVT as demonstrated by a global CASQ2 KO model [20], this result argues against Purkinje cells as the origin of CPVT, at least not on their own. On the other hand, in support of myocytes as the origin of CPVT, cells isolated from the myocardium of CPVT mouse models have been shown to exhibit DCR, DAD, and ectopic action potentials in multiple studies [20, 66, 67, 80]. Human iPSC-derived cardiomyocytes generated from biopsies of human CPVT patients also displayed DCR, DAD, and ectopic action potentials characteristic of the above-mentioned CPVT cells [84, 85]. Drug studies based on isolated myocytes also serve as good indicators of drug efficacy in both mouse models and humans [22, 86, 87]. More evidence regarding the cellular origin of CPVT are discussed elsewhere [22].

9. Therapies for CPVT

Symptoms of CPVT vary from palpitations, syncope, or even cardiac arrest. Although a rare disease, the mortality rate of CPVT can reach as high as ~50% in untreated individuals before the age of 40 [23]. In this section, we will first discuss traditional therapies that are currently available to CPVT patients. Next, we will focus on novel therapeutic approaches, based on recent advances in understanding the molecular mechanisms of this life-threatening arrhythmia syndrome.

9.1 Current therapies for CPVT

9.1.1 Beta-blockers

Beta-blockers are the first-line drug therapy to treat CPVT. As discussed above, in CPVT, the β-adrenergic-dependent increase in SR Ca load is important in triggering DCR and subsequent cellular arrhythmogenesis. Thus, blocking the β-adrenergic signaling pathway is expected to decrease DCR and suppress arrhythmias. The most effective beta-blocker at the time of writing is nadolol [88, 89], but it remains unknown why it is more effective than other beta-blockers. Unfortunately, beta-blockers only offer limited protection even with the maximal tolerated dose. It has been reported that more than 30% patients still suffer from arrhythmic events after receiving beta-blockers [90].

Carvedilol, a beta-blocker that is highly effective in preventing VT in heart failure, has been shown to suppress CPVT through a dual inhibitory action on both β-adrenergic signaling and RyR2 channel activity [91]. Experimentally, an analog of carvedilol with minimal beta-blocking activity still prevented VT in a CPVT mouse model and exhibited improved efficacy when combined with a selective beta-blocker [91]. Nevertheless, further studies are required to assess its effectiveness in CPVT patients. However, this provides a new potential pharmacological approach where a combination of RyR2 channel inhibition and beta-blockade could provide a more effective therapeutic approach than current options based solely on beta-blockers.

9.1.2 Na channel blockers and flecainide

Na channel blockers may serve as anti-arrhythmic drugs due to the critical role of the Nav 1.5 channel in the depolarization phase of action potential. Flecainide, an FDA approved drug to treat arrhythmias, was originally thought to work by blocking the Na channel. Recent studies have found that flecainide prevents CPVT both in mouse models and human patients through a dual inhibition mechanism: inhibiting Na channels as well as RyR2 [86]. Studies show that flecainide appears to be a promising therapy for CPVT patients not responding well to beta-blockers. However, the working mechanism of flecainide was controversial.

A study conducted on the CPVT model of RyR2 R4496C$^{+/-}$ showed that while flecainide was effective in preventing arrhythmias, it did not reduce DCR in the cellular experiments. Instead, it increased the threshold for triggered activity, thus pointing to the other possibility: that the drug works by solely acting as a Na channel blocker [92]. Several follow-up studies attempted to reconcile this discrepancy. Evidence has been provided that flecainide is effective in reducing DCR in cells harboring the RyR2 R4496C$^{+/-}$ mutation, but this effect could be masked by experimental conditions such as Ca overload [93]. On the other hand, more convincing evidence comes from a recent study that employed a synthesized analog of flecainide with reduced inhibition on RyR2 activity but unaltered inhibition on Na channel [94]. This analog failed to reduce DCR at cellular level and arrhythmia burden *in vivo,* indicating that flecainide acts through inhibition of RyR2 activity. In support of this, flecainide reduced DCR in permeabilized CPVT cells lacking membrane-residing Na channels, and intact cells pretreated with Na channel blocker. Similar to flecainide, another approved drug propafenone also seems to work through dual inhibition of Na channel and RyR2 [95]. Further studies are required to fully understand its working mechanism.

9.1.3 Other treatment options

Ca channel blockers (LTCC blockers) such as verapamil, have been tested in cellular and animal studies, as well as clinical studies, to examine their efficacy in treating CPVT. Consistently, these studies found Ca channel blockers only confer limited benefits in both cellular preparations and patients already on beta-blockers [96–98]. However, it has been shown to be beneficial for some patients when used in combination with other pharmacological approaches including beta-blockers [98].

Left cardiac sympathetic denervation serves as an alternative treatment. It works by preventing the release of catecholamines from the sympathetic nerve endings. The procedure appears to be effective in reducing major arrhythmic events in clinical studies [99, 100], and thus has been recommended for patients who don't respond to more conventional pharmacological treatments such as beta-blocker therapy. In one case employing an extrapleural approach, the lower part of the stellate ganglion was ablated together with the second and third thoracic ganglia [99]; another case used the thoracoscopic, the transaxillary, and the supraclavicular approaches as the main surgical approaches [100].

Implantable cardiac defibrillators (ICD) have been utilized in patients who still experience symptoms despite drug therapy and/or sympathetic denervation. A recent study systematically analyzed the efficacy of ICDs using existing clinical data containing 505 CPVT patients implanted with ICDs [101]. It was found that although effective for ventricular fibrillation, ICDs were not protective for VT. Another study of 136 CPVT patients also suggests ICD implant did not confer survival benefits [102]. Considering the potential complications and psychological burden of implantation, especially for pediatric patients, ICDs are not an optimal treatment for CPVT patients.

9.2 Potential future therapies for CPVT

The molecular mechanisms underlying CPVT have been intensively studied in the past several decades. Several novel therapeutic strategies have been proposed and tested in animal models and even pre-clinical studies. In this section, we will discuss these novel approaches, with a focus on gene therapy.

9.2.1 Gene therapy

With advances in the adeno-associated virus (AAV) vector-based gene transfer technology in the past a few decades, using gene therapy to treat CPVT is starting to become technically feasible. Several proof-of-principle studies have been conducted to test the efficacy of different therapeutic strategies. Considering several CPVT mutations, especially the ones identified in CASQ2, cause loss or reduced expression of the associated protein, it would seem that the most straightforward therapeutic approach is to deliver a normal gene encoding the protein. Indeed, AAV9-mediated gene transfer of a WT CASQ2 to both CASQ2 KO and R33Q mouse models restored the normal expression of CASQ2, improved abnormal electrophysiological properties of cells, and reduced arrhythmia burden *in vivo* [103, 104]. However, this gene replacement approach is limited by the size of the AAV vector, thus hindering the delivery of a normal gene for the large RyR2 protein, which accounts for the majority of the CPVT mutations. To solve this problem, AAV9 was instead used to deliver siRNA to silence mutant mRNA of RyR2 in an allele-specific way [105]. This RNA silencing approach increased the ratio of WT-RNA vs. mutant RNA, proving to be effective at normalizing cardiac electrophysiology, alleviating abnormal ultrastructural remodeling, and inhibiting *in vivo* VT when tested in the RyR2 R4496C$^{+/-}$ mice. Alternatively, another study attempted *in vivo* genome editing using the CRISPR/Cas9 system delivered by AAV and also obtained promising results in a different CPVT model of RyR2 (R176Q$^{+/-}$) [106].

While theses gene therapy strategies seem effective, one of the prerequisites for applying this technology is knowing the genetic cause of CPVT. However, the genetic cause of ~30–40% of clinical cases of CPVT remains undetermined. Several groups have developed novel approaches to tackle this problem. It has been found that the Ca binding properties of CaM—in particular, the kinetics of Ca dissociation from CaM—affects RyR2 refractoriness [66]. Based on this, a therapeutic CaM (TCaM) that specifically targets RyR2 and prolongs its refractoriness by slowing Ca dissociation from CaM was engineered. TCaM reduced DCR in CPVT cells and alleviated arrhythmias *in vivo* when delivered to a CPVT model of CASQ2 R33Q mice [66]. Instead of targeting the specific disease-causing gene, TCaM targets the impaired RyR2 refractoriness, and thus it could potentially serve as a therapeutic avenue for distinct forms of CPVT. Another study chose to target CaMKII, an adrenergically activated kinase that is implicated in arrhythmogenesis and pathological remodeling in multiple cardiac disorders, including CPVT. Pharmacological inhibitors of CaMKII are limited in their efficacy due to their lack of specificity. In contrast, a CaMKII inhibitory peptide was delivered in a cardiomyocyte-specific way by AAV9 and found to be effective in reducing arrhythmias burden *in vivo* in the CPVT model of RyR2 ($R176Q^{+/-}$) [107]. Collectively, these studies provide strong evidence supporting AAV-based gene therapy as a promising future therapy for CPVT patients.

9.3 Targeting sinus node dysfunction

CPVT patients also present sinus node dysfunction and bradycardia, which are recapitulated in the mouse models of CPVT. The pathophysiological role and underlying mechanism for sinus node dysfunction are discussed in details elsewhere [22]. Targeting the impaired sinus node dysfunction has been proposed as a therapeutic approach for CPVT. It has been shown that increasing heart rate by (1) pharmacological intervention (atropine), (2) atrial overdrive pacing, or (3) re-expressing CASQ2 in the CASQ2 KO mouse all appear to reduce arrhythmia burden [83, 108]. Further, atropine has been tested in a small group of 6 CPVT patients and was found to be effective in reducing exercise-induced arrhythmic events [109].

9.4 Other potential therapies

Tremendous effort has been expended on identifying and developing small molecules that specifically target DCR of RyR2, since DCR is implicated in a spectrum of cardiac disorders. Dantrolene, a drug used clinically to treat a skeletal muscle condition of malignant hyperthermia, exhibited partial protection for a subset of CPVT patients [110]. The recently discovered ent-(+)-verticilide, an unnatural verticilide enantiomer, appears to be a potent and selective RyR2 inhibitor [87]. It reduced DCR, triggered activity in cells, and arrhythmias *in vivo* when tested with the CPVT model of CASQ2 KO. It seems to exert a stronger antiarrhythmic effect when compared with dantrolene or flecainide. More details on the current state of therapeutic small molecule development are reviewed elsewhere [111].

10. Conclusion

Great progress has been made in the past few decades to help us better understand CPVT and develop therapeutics for this deadly arrhythmia syndrome. These efforts will continue in both basic science and clinical studies and will provide deeper mechanistic insight on the molecular, cellular, and tissue mechanisms of CPVT. Since DCR is implicated in a spectrum of human diseases, knowledge obtained from these studies will also benefit the development of therapies for other cardiac dysfunctions including heart failure and metabolic heart disease.

Acknowledgements

We want to thank the American Heart Association for providing funding and National Institutes of Health (1R15HL154073).

Abbreviation list

AAV	adeno-associated virus
Ca	calcium
CALM	calmodulin (gene)
CaM	calmodulin (protein)
CASQ2	calsequestrin 2
CICR	calcium-induced calcium release
CPVT	catecholaminergic polymorphic ventricular tachycardia
DAD	delayed afterdepolarization
DCR	dysregulated calcium release
DKO	double knockout
EAD	early afterdepolarization
ECC	excitation-contraction coupling
HEK29	human embryonic kidney cells
HRC	histidine-rich calcium binding protein
ICD	implantable cardiac defibrillators
iPSC	induced pluripotent stem cells
LTCC	L-type calcium channel
PLN	phospholamban
RyR2	type 2 ryanodine receptor
NCX	sodium calcium exchanger
SERCA	sarcoplasmic reticulum calcium ATPase
SOICR	store-overload-induced calcium release
SR	sarcoplasmic reticulum
TCaM	therapeutic calmodulin
TRDN	triadin
VT	ventricular tachycardia

Author details

Bin Liu[1]*, Brian D. Tow[1] and Ingrid M. Bonilla[2]

1 Department of Biological Sciences, Mississippi State University, Starkville, Mississippi, USA

2 Department of Pharmacology and Toxicology, University of Puerto Rico Medical School, San Juan, Puerto Rico, USA

*Address all correspondence to: bl1190@msstate.edu

References

[1] Bers DM. Cardiac excitation-contraction coupling. Nature. 2002;415(6868):198-205.

[2] Gyorke S, Carnes C. Dysregulated sarcoplasmic reticulum calcium release: potential pharmacological target in cardiac disease. Pharmacol Ther. 2008;119(3):340-54.

[3] Belevych AE, Radwanski PB, Carnes CA, Gyorke S. 'Ryanopathy': causes and manifestations of RyR2 dysfunction in heart failure. Cardiovascular research. 2013;98(2):240-7.

[4] Gyorke S. Molecular basis of catecholaminergic polymorphic ventricular tachycardia. Heart Rhythm. 2009;6(1):123-9.

[5] Priori SG, Chen SR. Inherited dysfunction of sarcoplasmic reticulum Ca2+ handling and arrhythmogenesis. Circulation research. 2011;108(7):871-83.

[6] Scriven DR, Asghari P, Moore ED. Microarchitecture of the dyad. Cardiovascular research. 2013;98(2):169-76.

[7] Cheng H, Lederer WJ, Cannell MB. Calcium sparks: elementary events underlying excitation-contraction coupling in heart muscle. Science. 1993;262(5134):740-4.

[8] Bassani JW, Bassani RA, Bers DM. Twitch-dependent SR Ca accumulation and release in rabbit ventricular myocytes. Am J Physiol. 1993;265(2 Pt 1):C533-40.

[9] Shannon TR, Guo T, Bers DM. Ca2+ scraps: local depletions of free [Ca2+] in cardiac sarcoplasmic reticulum during contractions leave substantial Ca2+ reserve. Circulation research. 2003;93(1):40-5.

[10] Fabiato A. Time and calcium dependence of activation and inactivation of calcium-induced release of calcium from the sarcoplasmic reticulum of a skinned canine cardiac Purkinje cell. The Journal of general physiology. 1985;85(2):247-89.

[11] Gyorke I, Gyorke S. Regulation of the cardiac ryanodine receptor channel by luminal Ca2+ involves luminal Ca2+ sensing sites. Biophysical journal. 1998;75(6):2801-10.

[12] Gyorke I, Hester N, Jones LR, Gyorke S. The role of calsequestrin, triadin, and junctin in conferring cardiac ryanodine receptor responsiveness to luminal calcium. Biophysical journal. 2004;86(4):2121-8.

[13] Terentyev D, Viatchenko-Karpinski S, Valdivia HH, Escobar AL, Gyorke S. Luminal Ca2+ controls termination and refractory behavior of Ca2+–induced Ca2+ release in cardiac myocytes. Circulation research. 2002;91(5):414-20.

[14] Sobie EA, Dilly KW, dos Santos Cruz J, Lederer WJ, Jafri MS. Termination of cardiac Ca(2+) sparks: an investigative mathematical model of calcium-induced calcium release. Biophysical journal. 2002;83(1):59-78.

[15] Jiang D, Xiao B, Yang D, Wang R, Choi P, Zhang L, et al. RyR2 mutations linked to ventricular tachycardia and sudden death reduce the threshold for store-overload-induced Ca2+ release (SOICR). Proceedings of the National Academy of Sciences of the United States of America. 2004;101(35):13062-7.

[16] Chen W, Wang R, Chen B, Zhong X, Kong H, Bai Y, et al. The ryanodine receptor store-sensing gate controls Ca2+ waves and Ca2+–triggered arrhythmias. Nature medicine. 2014;20(2):184-92.

[17] Peng W, Shen H, Wu J, Guo W, Pan X, Wang R, et al. Structural basis for the gating mechanism of the type 2 ryanodine receptor RyR2. Science. 2016;354(6310).

[18] Terentyev D, Viatchenko-Karpinski S, Gyorke I, Volpe P, Williams SC, Gyorke S. Calsequestrin determines the functional size and stability of cardiac intracellular calcium stores: Mechanism for hereditary arrhythmia. Proceedings of the National Academy of Sciences of the United States of America. 2003;100(20): 11759-64.

[19] Terentyev D, Viatchenko-Karpinski S, Vedamoorthyrao S, Oduru S, Gyorke I, Williams SC, et al. Protein protein interactions between triadin and calsequestrin are involved in modulation of sarcoplasmic reticulum calcium release in cardiac myocytes. The Journal of physiology. 2007;583 (Pt 1):71-80.

[20] Knollmann BC, Chopra N, Hlaing T, Akin B, Yang T, Ettensohn K, et al. Casq2 deletion causes sarcoplasmic reticulum volume increase, premature Ca2+ release, and catecholaminergic polymorphic ventricular tachycardia. The Journal of clinical investigation. 2006;116(9):2510-20.

[21] Liu B, Ho HT, Brunello L, Unudurthi SD, Lou Q, Belevych AE, et al. Ablation of HRC alleviates cardiac arrhythmia and improves abnormal Ca handling in CASQ2 knockout mice prone to CPVT. Cardiovascular research. 2015;108(2):299-311.

[22] Wleklinski MJ, Kannankeril PJ, Knollmann BC. Molecular and tissue mechanisms of catecholaminergic polymorphic ventricular tachycardia. The Journal of physiology. 2020;598(14): 2817-34.

[23] Perez-Riera AR, Barbosa-Barros R, de Rezende Barbosa MPC, Daminello-Raimundo R, de Lucca AA, Jr., de Abreu LC. Catecholaminergic polymorphic ventricular tachycardia, an update. Ann Noninvasive Electrocardiol. 2018;23(4):e12512.

[24] Roston TM, Yuchi Z, Kannankeril PJ, Hathaway J, Vinocur JM, Etheridge SP, et al. The clinical and genetic spectrum of catecholaminergic polymorphic ventricular tachycardia: findings from an international multicentre registry. Europace. 2018;20(3):541-7.

[25] Roston TM, Sanatani S, Chen SR. Suppression-of-function mutations in the cardiac ryanodine receptor: Emerging evidence for a novel arrhythmia syndrome? Heart Rhythm. 2017;14(1):108-9.

[26] Zhao YT, Valdivia CR, Gurrola GB, Powers PP, Willis BC, Moss RL, et al. Arrhythmogenesis in a catecholaminergic polymorphic ventricular tachycardia mutation that depresses ryanodine receptor function. Proceedings of the National Academy of Sciences of the United States of America. 2015;112(13):E1669-77.

[27] Kujala K, Paavola J, Lahti A, Larsson K, Pekkanen-Mattila M, Viitasalo M, et al. Cell model of catecholaminergic polymorphic ventricular tachycardia reveals early and delayed afterdepolarizations. PLoS One. 2012;7(9):e44660.

[28] Wehrens XH, Lehnart SE, Huang F, Vest JA, Reiken SR, Mohler PJ, et al. FKBP12.6 deficiency and defective calcium release channel (ryanodine receptor) function linked to exercise-induced sudden cardiac death. Cell. 2003;113(7):829-40.

[29] Jiang D, Wang R, Xiao B, Kong H, Hunt DJ, Choi P, et al. Enhanced store overload-induced Ca2+ release and channel sensitivity to luminal Ca2+ activation are common defects of RyR2

mutations linked to ventricular tachycardia and sudden death. Circulation research. 2005;97(11): 1173-81.

[30] Liu N, Colombi B, Memmi M, Zissimopoulos S, Rizzi N, Negri S, et al. Arrhythmogenesis in catecholaminergic polymorphic ventricular tachycardia: insights from a RyR2 R4496C knock-in mouse model. Circulation research. 2006;99(3):292-8.

[31] George CH, Higgs GV, Lai FA. Ryanodine receptor mutations associated with stress-induced ventricular tachycardia mediate increased calcium release in stimulated cardiomyocytes. Circulation research. 2003;93(6):531-40.

[32] Zhang JZ, Waddell HM, Wu E, Dholakia J, Okolo CA, McLay JC, et al. FKBPs facilitate the termination of spontaneous Ca2+ release in wild-type RyR2 but not CPVT mutant RyR2. Biochem J. 2016;473(14):2049-60.

[33] Yano M, Yamamoto T, Ikemoto N, Matsuzaki M. Abnormal ryanodine receptor function in heart failure. Pharmacol Ther. 2005;107(3):377-91.

[34] George CH, Jundi H, Thomas NL, Fry DL, Lai FA. Ryanodine receptors and ventricular arrhythmias: emerging trends in mutations, mechanisms and therapies. Journal of molecular and cellular cardiology. 2007;42(1):34-50.

[35] Ikemoto N, Yamamoto T. Regulation of calcium release by interdomain interaction within ryanodine receptors. Front Biosci. 2002;7:d671-83.

[36] George CH, Jundi H, Walters N, Thomas NL, West RR, Lai FA. Arrhythmogenic mutation-linked defects in ryanodine receptor autoregulation reveal a novel mechanism of Ca2+ release channel dysfunction. Circulation research. 2006;98(1):88-97.

[37] Sumitomo N. Current topics in catecholaminergic polymorphic ventricular tachycardia. J Arrhythm. 2016;32(5):344-51.

[38] Gray B, Bagnall RD, Lam L, Ingles J, Turner C, Haan E, et al. A novel heterozygous mutation in cardiac calsequestrin causes autosomal dominant catecholaminergic polymorphic ventricular tachycardia. Heart Rhythm. 2016;13(8):1652-60.

[39] Scott BT, Simmerman HK, Collins JH, Nadal-Ginard B, Jones LR. Complete amino acid sequence of canine cardiac calsequestrin deduced by cDNA cloning. The Journal of biological chemistry. 1988;263(18):8958-64.

[40] Yano K, Zarain-Herzberg A. Sarcoplasmic reticulum calsequestrins: structural and functional properties. Mol Cell Biochem. 1994;135(1):61-70.

[41] Park H, Park IY, Kim E, Youn B, Fields K, Dunker AK, et al. Comparing skeletal and cardiac calsequestrin structures and their calcium binding: a proposed mechanism for coupled calcium binding and protein polymerization. The Journal of biological chemistry. 2004;279(17): 18026-33.

[42] Gyorke S, Terentyev D. Modulation of ryanodine receptor by luminal calcium and accessory proteins in health and cardiac disease. Cardiovascular research. 2008;77(2):245-55.

[43] Terentyev D, Kubalova Z, Valle G, Nori A, Vedamoorthyrao S, Terentyeva R, et al. Modulation of SR Ca release by luminal Ca and calsequestrin in cardiac myocytes: effects of CASQ2 mutations linked to sudden cardiac death. Biophysical journal. 2008;95(4):2037-48.

[44] Manno C, Figueroa LC, Gillespie D, Fitts R, Kang C, Franzini-Armstrong C, et al. Calsequestrin depolymerizes when

calcium is depleted in the sarcoplasmic reticulum of working muscle. Proceedings of the National Academy of Sciences of the United States of America. 2017;114(4):E638-E47.

[45] Terentyev D, Nori A, Santoro M, Viatchenko-Karpinski S, Kubalova Z, Gyorke I, et al. Abnormal interactions of calsequestrin with the ryanodine receptor calcium release channel complex linked to exercise-induced sudden cardiac death. Circulation research. 2006;98(9):1151-8.

[46] Dirksen WP, Lacombe VA, Chi M, Kalyanasundaram A, Viatchenko-Karpinski S, Terentyev D, et al. A mutation in calsequestrin, CASQ2D307H, impairs Sarcoplasmic Reticulum Ca2+ handling and causes complex ventricular arrhythmias in mice. Cardiovascular research. 2007;75(1):69-78.

[47] Titus EW, Deiter FH, Shi C, Wojciak J, Scheinman M, Jura N, et al. The structure of a calsequestrin filament reveals mechanisms of familial arrhythmia. Nat Struct Mol Biol. 2020;27(12):1142-51.

[48] Kobayashi YM, Alseikhan BA, Jones LR. Localization and characterization of the calsequestrin-binding domain of triadin 1. Evidence for a charged beta-strand in mediating the protein-protein interaction. The Journal of biological chemistry. 2000;275(23):17639-46.

[49] Kirchhefer U, Neumann J, Baba HA, Begrow F, Kobayashi YM, Reinke U, et al. Cardiac hypertrophy and impaired relaxation in transgenic mice overexpressing triadin 1. The Journal of biological chemistry. 2001;276(6): 4142-9.

[50] Chopra N, Yang T, Asghari P, Moore ED, Huke S, Akin B, et al. Ablation of triadin causes loss of cardiac Ca2+ release units, impaired excitation-contraction coupling, and cardiac arrhythmias. Proceedings of the National Academy of Sciences of the United States of America. 2009;106(18):7636-41.

[51] Terentyev D, Cala SE, Houle TD, Viatchenko-Karpinski S, Gyorke I, Terentyeva R, et al. Triadin overexpression stimulates excitation-contraction coupling and increases predisposition to cellular arrhythmia in cardiac myocytes. Circulation research. 2005;96(6):651-8.

[52] Roux-Buisson N, Cacheux M, Fourest-Lieuvin A, Fauconnier J, Brocard J, Denjoy I, et al. Absence of triadin, a protein of the calcium release complex, is responsible for cardiac arrhythmia with sudden death in human. Hum Mol Genet. 2012;21(12): 2759-67.

[53] Rooryck C, Kyndt F, Bozon D, Roux-Buisson N, Sacher F, Probst V, et al. New Family With Catecholaminergic Polymorphic Ventricular Tachycardia Linked to the Triadin Gene. J Cardiovasc Electrophysiol. 2015;26(10):1146-50.

[54] Linse S, Helmersson A, Forsen S. Calcium binding to calmodulin and its globular domains. The Journal of biological chemistry. 1991;266(13): 8050-4.

[55] VanScyoc WS, Sorensen BR, Rusinova E, Laws WR, Ross JB, Shea MA. Calcium binding to calmodulin mutants monitored by domain-specific intrinsic phenylalanine and tyrosine fluorescence. Biophysical journal. 2002;83(5):2767-80.

[56] Yamniuk AP, Vogel HJ. Calmodulin's flexibility allows for promiscuity in its interactions with target proteins and peptides. Mol Biotechnol. 2004;27(1): 33-57.

[57] Yang Y, Guo T, Oda T, Chakraborty A, Chen L, Uchinoumi H,

et al. Cardiac myocyte Z-line calmodulin is mainly RyR2-bound, and reduction is arrhythmogenic and occurs in heart failure. Circulation research. 2014;114(2):295-306.

[58] Yamaguchi N, Xu L, Pasek DA, Evans KE, Meissner G. Molecular basis of calmodulin binding to cardiac muscle Ca(2+) release channel (ryanodine receptor). The Journal of biological chemistry. 2003;278(26):23480-6.

[59] Hwang HS, Nitu FR, Yang Y, Walweel K, Pereira L, Johnson CN, et al. Divergent regulation of ryanodine receptor 2 calcium release channels by arrhythmogenic human calmodulin missense mutants. Circulation research. 2014;114(7):1114-24.

[60] Gyorke S, Belevych AE, Liu B, Kubasov IV, Carnes CA, Radwanski PB. The role of luminal Ca regulation in Ca signaling refractoriness and cardiac arrhythmogenesis. The Journal of general physiology. 2017;149(9):877-88.

[61] DelPrincipe F, Egger M, Niggli E. Calcium signalling in cardiac muscle: refractoriness revealed by coherent activation. Nat Cell Biol. 1999;1(6): 323-9.

[62] Szentesi P, Pignier C, Egger M, Kranias EG, Niggli E. Sarcoplasmic reticulum Ca2+ refilling controls recovery from Ca2+–induced Ca2+ release refractoriness in heart muscle. Circulation research. 2004;95(8):807-13.

[63] Belevych AE, Terentyev D, Terentyeva R, Ho HT, Gyorke I, Bonilla IM, et al. Shortened Ca2+ signaling refractoriness underlies cellular arrhythmogenesis in a postinfarction model of sudden cardiac death. Circulation research. 2012;110(4):569-77.

[64] Kornyeyev D, Petrosky AD, Zepeda B, Ferreiro M, Knollmann B, Escobar AL. Calsequestrin 2 deletion shortens the refractoriness of Ca(2)(+) release and reduces rate-dependent Ca(2)(+)-alternans in intact mouse hearts. Journal of molecular and cellular cardiology. 2012;52(1):21-31.

[65] Brunello L, Slabaugh JL, Radwanski PB, Ho HT, Belevych AE, Lou Q, et al. Decreased RyR2 refractoriness determines myocardial synchronization of aberrant Ca2+ release in a genetic model of arrhythmia. Proceedings of the National Academy of Sciences of the United States of America. 2013;110(25): 10312-7.

[66] Liu B, Walton SD, Ho HT, Belevych AE, Tikunova SB, Bonilla I, et al. Gene Transfer of Engineered Calmodulin Alleviates Ventricular Arrhythmias in a Calsequestrin-Associated Mouse Model of Catecholaminergic Polymorphic Ventricular Tachycardia. Journal of the American Heart Association. 2018;7(10).

[67] Loaiza R, Benkusky NA, Powers PP, Hacker T, Noujaim S, Ackerman MJ, et al. Heterogeneity of ryanodine receptor dysfunction in a mouse model of catecholaminergic polymorphic ventricular tachycardia. Circulation research. 2013;112(2):298-308.

[68] Lakatta EG. Functional implications of spontaneous sarcoplasmic reticulum Ca2+ release in the heart. Cardiovascular research. 1992;26(3):193-214.

[69] Marban E, Robinson SW, Wier WG. Mechanisms of arrhythmogenic delayed and early afterdepolarizations in ferret ventricular muscle. The Journal of clinical investigation. 1986;78(5): 1185-92.

[70] Orchard CH, Eisner DA, Allen DG. Oscillations of intracellular Ca2+ in mammalian cardiac muscle. Nature. 1983;304(5928):735-8.

[71] Pogwizd SM, Bers DM. Cellular basis of triggered arrhythmias in heart failure. Trends Cardiovasc Med. 2004;14(2):61-6.

[72] Schlotthauer K, Bers DM. Sarcoplasmic reticulum Ca(2+) release causes myocyte depolarization. Underlying mechanism and threshold for triggered action potentials. Circulation research. 2000;87(9): 774-80.

[73] Hoeker GS, Katra RP, Wilson LD, Plummer BN, Laurita KR. Spontaneous calcium release in tissue from the failing canine heart. Am J Physiol Heart Circ Physiol. 2009;297(4):H1235-42.

[74] Kalyanasundaram A, Lacombe VA, Belevych AE, Brunello L, Carnes CA, Janssen PM, et al. Up-regulation of sarcoplasmic reticulum Ca(2+) uptake leads to cardiac hypertrophy, contractile dysfunction and early mortality in mice deficient in CASQ2. Cardiovascular research. 2013;98(2):297-306.

[75] Liu B, Lou Q, Smith H, Velez-Cortes F, Dillmann WH, Knollmann BC, et al. Conditional Up-Regulation of SERCA2a Exacerbates RyR2-Dependent Ventricular and Atrial Arrhythmias. Int J Mol Sci. 2020;21(7).

[76] Bai Y, Jones PP, Guo J, Zhong X, Clark RB, Zhou Q, et al. Phospholamban knockout breaks arrhythmogenic Ca(2)(+) waves and suppresses catecho laminergic polymorphic ventricular tachycardia in mice. Circulation research. 2013;113(5):517-26.

[77] Valverde CA, Mazzocchi G, Di Carlo MN, Ciocci Pardo A, Salas N, Ragone MI, et al. Ablation of phospholamban rescues reperfusion arrhythmias but exacerbates myocardium infarction in hearts with Ca2+/calmodulin kinase II constitutive phosphorylation of ryanodine receptors. Cardiovascular research. 2019;115(3):556-69.

[78] Xie Y, Sato D, Garfinkel A, Qu Z, Weiss JN. So little source, so much sink: requirements for afterdepolarizations to propagate in tissue. Biophysical journal. 2010;99(5):1408-15.

[79] Sommer JR, Johnson EA. Cardiac muscle. A comparative study of Purkinje fibers and ventricular fibers. J Cell Biol. 1968;36(3):497-526.

[80] Cerrone M, Noujaim SF, Tolkacheva EG, Talkachou A, O'Connell R, Berenfeld O, et al. Arrhythmogenic mechanisms in a mouse model of catecholaminergic polymorphic ventricular tachycardia. Circulation research. 2007;101(10): 1039-48.

[81] Herron TJ, Milstein ML, Anumonwo J, Priori SG, Jalife J. Purkinje cell calcium dysregulation is the cellular mechanism that underlies catecholaminergic polymorphic ventricular tachycardia. Heart Rhythm. 2010;7(8):1122-8.

[82] Kang G, Giovannone SF, Liu N, Liu FY, Zhang J, Priori SG, et al. Purkinje cells from RyR2 mutant mice are highly arrhythmogenic but responsive to targeted therapy. Circulation research. 2010;107(4):512-9.

[83] Flores DJ, Duong T, Bran denberger LO, Mitra A, Shirali A, Johnson JC, et al. Conditional ablation and conditional rescue models for Casq2 elucidate the role of development and of cell-type specific expression of Casq2 in the CPVT2 phenotype. Hum Mol Genet. 2018;27(9):1533-44.

[84] Novak A, Barad L, Lorber A, Gherghiceanu M, Reiter I, Eisen B, et al. Functional abnormalities in iPSC-derived cardiomyocytes generated from CPVT1 and CPVT2 patients carrying ryanodine or calsequestrin mutations. J Cell Mol Med. 2015;19(8):2006-18.

[85] Novak A, Barad L, Zeevi-Levin N, Shick R, Shtrichman R, Lorber A, et al.

Cardiomyocytes generated from CPVTD307H patients are arrhythmogenic in response to beta-adrenergic stimulation. J Cell Mol Med. 2012;16(3):468-82.

[86] Watanabe H, Chopra N, Laver D, Hwang HS, Davies SS, Roach DE, et al. Flecainide prevents catecholaminergic polymorphic ventricular tachycardia in mice and humans. Nature medicine. 2009;15(4):380-3.

[87] Batiste SM, Blackwell DJ, Kim K, Kryshtal DO, Gomez-Hurtado N, Rebbeck RT, et al. Unnatural verticilide enantiomer inhibits type 2 ryanodine receptor-mediated calcium leak and is antiarrhythmic. Proceedings of the National Academy of Sciences of the United States of America. 2019;116(11): 4810-5.

[88] Hayashi M, Denjoy I, Extramiana F, Maltret A, Buisson NR, Lupoglazoff JM, et al. Incidence and risk factors of arrhythmic events in catecholaminergic polymorphic ventricular tachycardia. Circulation. 2009;119(18):2426-34.

[89] Leren IS, Saberniak J, Majid E, Haland TF, Edvardsen T, Haugaa KH. Nadolol decreases the incidence and severity of ventricular arrhythmias during exercise stress testing compared with beta1-selective beta-blockers in patients with catecholaminergic polymorphic ventricular tachycardia. Heart Rhythm. 2016;13(2): 433-40.

[90] van der Werf C, Zwinderman AH, Wilde AA. Therapeutic approach for patients with catecholaminergic polymorphic ventricular tachycardia: state of the art and future developments. Europace. 2012;14(2):175-83.

[91] Zhou Q, Xiao J, Jiang D, Wang R, Vembaiyan K, Wang A, et al. Carvedilol and its new analogs suppress arrhythmogenic store overload-induced Ca2+ release. Nature medicine. 2011;17(8):1003-9.

[92] Liu N, Denegri M, Ruan Y, Avelino-Cruz JE, Perissi A, Negri S, et al. Short communication: flecainide exerts an antiarrhythmic effect in a mouse model of catecholaminergic polymorphic ventricular tachycardia by increasing the threshold for triggered activity. Circulation research. 2011;109(3):291-5.

[93] Hwang HS, Baldo MP, Rodriguez JP, Faggioni M, Knollmann BC. Efficacy of Flecainide in Catecholaminergic Polymorphic Ventricular Tachycardia Is Mutation-Independent but Reduced by Calcium Overload. Front Physiol. 2019;10:992.

[94] Kryshtal DO, Blackwell DJ, Egly CL, Smith AN, Batiste SM, Johnston JN, et al. RYR2 Channel Inhibition Is the Principal Mechanism of Flecainide Action in CPVT. Circulation research. 2021;128(3):321-31.

[95] Hwang HS, Hasdemir C, Laver D, Mehra D, Turhan K, Faggioni M, et al. Inhibition of cardiac Ca2+ release channels (RyR2) determines efficacy of class I antiarrhythmic drugs in catecholaminergic polymorphic ventricular tachycardia. Circ Arrhythm Electrophysiol. 2011;4(2): 128-35.

[96] Swan H, Laitinen P, Kontula K, Toivonen L. Calcium channel antagonism reduces exercise-induced ventricular arrhythmias in catecholaminergic polymorphic ventricular tachycardia patients with RyR2 mutations. J Cardiovasc Electrophysiol. 2005;16(2):162-6.

[97] Katz G, Khoury A, Kurtzwald E, Hochhauser E, Porat E, Shainberg A, et al. Optimizing catecholaminergic polymorphic ventricular tachycardia therapy in calsequestrin-mutant mice. Heart Rhythm. 2010;7(11):1676-82.

[98] Rosso R, Kalman JM, Rogowski O, Diamant S, Birger A, Biner S, et al. Calcium channel blockers and beta-blockers versus beta-blockers alone for preventing exercise-induced arrhythmias in catecholaminergic polymorphic ventricular tachycardia. Heart Rhythm. 2007;4(9):1149-54.

[99] Wilde AA, Bhuiyan ZA, Crotti L, Facchini M, De Ferrari GM, Paul T, et al. Left cardiac sympathetic denervation for catecholaminergic polymorphic ventricular tachycardia. N Engl J Med. 2008;358(19):2024-9.

[100] De Ferrari GM, Dusi V, Spazzolini C, Bos JM, Abrams DJ, Berul CI, et al. Clinical Management of Catecholaminergic Polymorphic Ventricular Tachycardia: The Role of Left Cardiac Sympathetic Denervation. Circulation. 2015;131(25):2185-93.

[101] Roston TM, Jones K, Hawkins NM, Bos JM, Schwartz PJ, Perry F, et al. Implantable cardioverter-defibrillator use in catecholaminergic polymorphic ventricular tachycardia: A systematic review. Heart Rhythm. 2018;15(12): 1791-9.

[102] van der Werf C, Lieve KV, Bos JM, Lane CM, Denjoy I, Roses-Noguer F, et al. Implantable cardioverter-defibrillators in previously undiagnosed patients with catecholaminergic polymorphic ventricular tachycardia resuscitated from sudden cardiac arrest. Eur Heart J. 2019;40(35):2953-61.

[103] Denegri M, Avelino-Cruz JE, Boncompagni S, De Simone SA, Auricchio A, Villani L, et al. Viral gene transfer rescues arrhythmogenic phenotype and ultrastructural abnormalities in adult calsequestrin-null mice with inherited arrhythmias. Circulation research. 2012;110(5):663-8.

[104] Denegri M, Bongianino R, Lodola F, Boncompagni S, De Giusti VC, Avelino-Cruz JE, et al. Single delivery of an adeno-associated viral construct to transfer the CASQ2 gene to knock-in mice affected by catecholaminergic polymorphic ventricular tachycardia is able to cure the disease from birth to advanced age. Circulation. 2014;129(25):2673-81.

[105] Bongianino R, Denegri M, Mazzanti A, Lodola F, Vollero A, Boncompagni S, et al. Allele-Specific Silencing of Mutant mRNA Rescues Ultrastructural and Arrhythmic Phenotype in Mice Carriers of the R4496C Mutation in the Ryanodine Receptor Gene (RYR2). Circulation research. 2017;121(5):525-36.

[106] Pan X, Philippen L, Lahiri SK, Lee C, Park SH, Word TA, et al. In Vivo Ryr2 Editing Corrects Catecholaminergic Polymorphic Ventricular Tachycardia. Circulation research. 2018;123(8):953-63.

[107] Bezzerides VJ, Caballero A, Wang S, Ai Y, Hylind RJ, Lu F, et al. Gene Therapy for Catecholaminergic Polymorphic Ventricular Tachycardia by Inhibition of Ca(2+)/Calmodulin-Dependent Kinase II. Circulation. 2019;140(5):405-19.

[108] Faggioni M, Hwang HS, van der Werf C, Nederend I, Kannankeril PJ, Wilde AA, et al. Accelerated sinus rhythm prevents catecholaminergic polymorphic ventricular tachycardia in mice and in patients. Circulation research. 2013;112(4):689-97.

[109] Kannankeril PJ, Shoemaker MB, Gayle KA, Fountain D, Roden DM, Knollmann BC. Atropine-induced sinus tachycardia protects against exercise-induced ventricular arrhythmias in patients with catecholaminergic polymorphic ventricular tachycardia. Europace. 2020;22(4):643-8.

[110] Penttinen K, Swan H, Vanninen S, Paavola J, Lahtinen AM, Kontula K, et al. Antiarrhythmic Effects of

Dantrolene in Patients with Catecholaminergic Polymorphic Ventricular Tachycardia and Replication of the Responses Using iPSC Models. PLoS One. 2015;10(5):e0125366.

[111] Connell P, Word TA, Wehrens XHT. Targeting pathological leak of ryanodine receptors: preclinical progress and the potential impact on treatments for cardiac arrhythmias and heart failure. Expert Opin Ther Targets. 2020;24(1):25-36.

Chapter 2

COVID-19 and Cardiac Enzymes

Meher Singha, Abhishek Madathanapalli and Raj Parikh

Abstract

Since December 2019, the COVID-19 pandemic has caused widespread mortality and adverse economic impact throughout the world. Though predominantly a respiratory disease, concerns regarding cardiovascular effects have been highlighted. Cardiac biomarkers and their elevations in COVID-19 have been associated with higher cardiovascular disease burden and worse prognosis. The mechanism of cardiac enzyme elevation in COVID-19 can be explained under two broad categories- direct injury caused by downregulation of ACE2 and hypoxemia, and indirect injury, which is mediated by the cytokine storm. Cardiac troponin and high sensitivity troponin are the most extensively studied cardiac enzymes in COVID-19. Studies have shown comparable and in some cases better predictive value than traditional markers of inflammation like d-dimer, C-reactive protein, lactate dehydrogenase. Natriuretic peptides such as BNP have utility as a robust prognostic marker in COVID-19 when considering outcomes like the need for mechanical ventilation and mortality. Emerging data from studies investigating the role of newer cardiac biomarkers in COVID-19 like mid-regional proadrenomedullin, growth differentiation factor-15 have also yielded promising results. As advances are made in our understanding of the pathogenesis, diagnosis, and management of COVID-19, it is evident that investigating the role of cardiac biomarkers in COVID-19 provides vital information.

Keywords: COVID-19, cardiac enzymes, COVID-19 infections, coronavirus, SARS-CoV-2, troponin, high sensitivity troponin, natriuretic peptides, creatine kinase, proadrenomedullin, growth differentiation factor-15, cardiac biomarkers, myocardial injury

1. Introduction

In December 2019, unexplained cases of pneumonia were reported from the epicenter of Wuhan City in China caused by a novel coronavirus, named severe acute respiratory syndrome coronavirus 2 (SARS-CoV-2). The transmissibility and virulence of this virus quickly transformed it into the worst global pandemic of our generation. The viral pneumonia syndrome was then named coronavirus disease 2019 (COVID-19) by World Health Organization. The COVID-19 pandemic continues to be a major cause of mortality and economic impact throughout the world. It is predominantly a respiratory disease, with a range of presentations varying from asymptomatic to severe respiratory failure. SARS-CoV-2 is known to enter human cells through angiotensin-converting enzyme 2, which is expressed not only in the lungs but also in other organs, such as the cardiovascular system, thus explaining the wide range of symptom manifestations. Significant concerns relating to

COVID-19 and the cardiovascular system have been highlighted, with COVID-19 inducing multiple cytokines and chemokines resulting in vascular inflammation, plaque instability, and myocardial inflammation. Several biomarkers have been studied that have related to COVID-19 progression as well as short-term mortality [1]. Cardiac biomarker and their elevation in COVID-19 have been studied and shown as a reflection of myocardial injury, hemodynamic stress, higher burden of cardiovascular disease, and worse prognosis [2]. Cardiac biomarkers have been suggested as possible aids for clinicians treating COVID-19 and understanding the severity of the disease and prognosis of patients. In this chapter, we will discuss the pathogenesis, role of specific cardiac biomarkers, and their use in the prognosis and management of COVID-19.

2. Epidemiology

The COVID-19 pandemic ranks as one of the most devastating events of the 21st century. Since 2019, the virus has spread rapidly across the globe with a reported case burden of upwards of 219 million with 4.5 million deaths. The United States of America, India, and Brazil reported the highest mortality among countries across the globe. The Centers for Disease Control and Prevention (CDC) estimates put the total number of COVID-19 cases in the United States at 44 million with 709,000 deaths. There is emerging data regarding the incidence and prevalence of cardiac injury in COVID-19 infection. Systematic reviews and meta-analyses have shown wide-ranging results. One meta-analysis demonstrated a 19% prevalence of cardiac injury in total COVID-19 cases, with 36% prevalence in severe cases, and 48% prevalence in non-survivors. Another meta-analysis showed a cardiac injury prevalence of 7.2% in total COVID-19 survivors, and 77% in non-survivors. While further analysis needs to be carried out to establish a more accurate prevalence of cardiac injury in COVID-19 infection, the prevalence of cardiac injury tends to increase along with the severity of the infection and poorer prognosis.

3. Pathogenesis

The pathobiology of elevation of cardiac enzymes in patients with COVID-19 can be divided into two major categories: (1) direct damage to the heart by down-regulation of ACE2, microvascular dysfunction, pericyte injury, and hypoxemia causing: myocarditis, heart failure, arrhythmias; and (2) indirect damage of cytokine storm by the release of cytokines, hyper inflammation, insulin resistance, coagulopathy causing: myocarditis, metabolic effect, thromboembolism. These are elucidated in **Figures 1** and **2**. Potential mechanisms of myocardial injury in COVID-19 include binding of the SARS-CoV2 virus to the endothelial angiotensin-converting enzyme 2 (ACE-2) receptor [3]. Given the low overall expression of angiotensin-converting enzyme 2 receptor in myocardial cells, the tropism of severe acute respiratory coronavirus 2 for the heart may be less likely. Myocardial injury has been reported in 36% patients hospitalized with COVID-19. Although clinical COVID-19 cases with myocardial injury and normal coronary arteries have been thought to be caused by myocarditis, ST-segment elevation myocardial infarctions (STEMI) may be caused by extensive microvascular thrombosis in the absence of epicardial coronary obstruction. On the other hand, indirect injury can occur as a consequence of a proinflammatory state, stress cardiomyopathy, and

DOI: http://dx.doi.org/10.5772/intechopen.101402

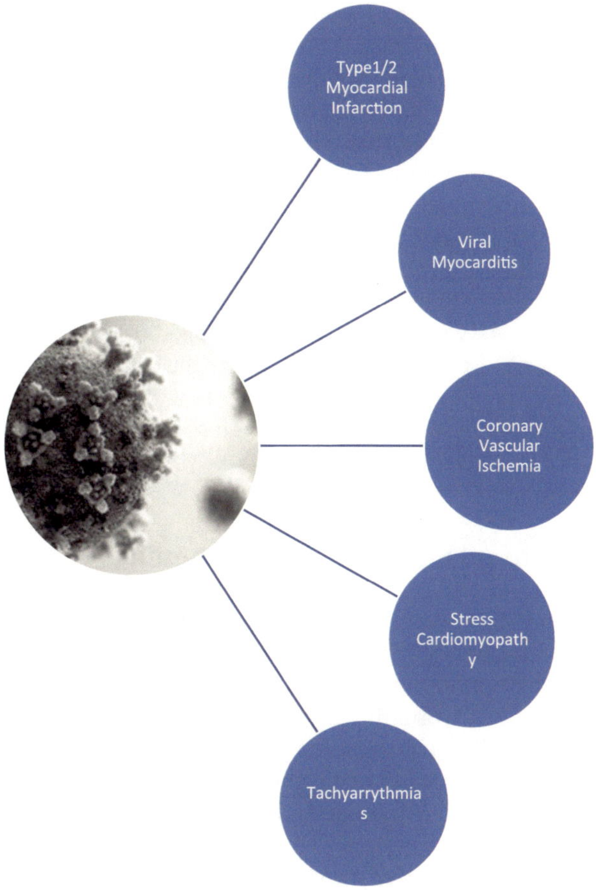

Figure 1.
Cardiac phenotypes of manifestations of COVID-19.

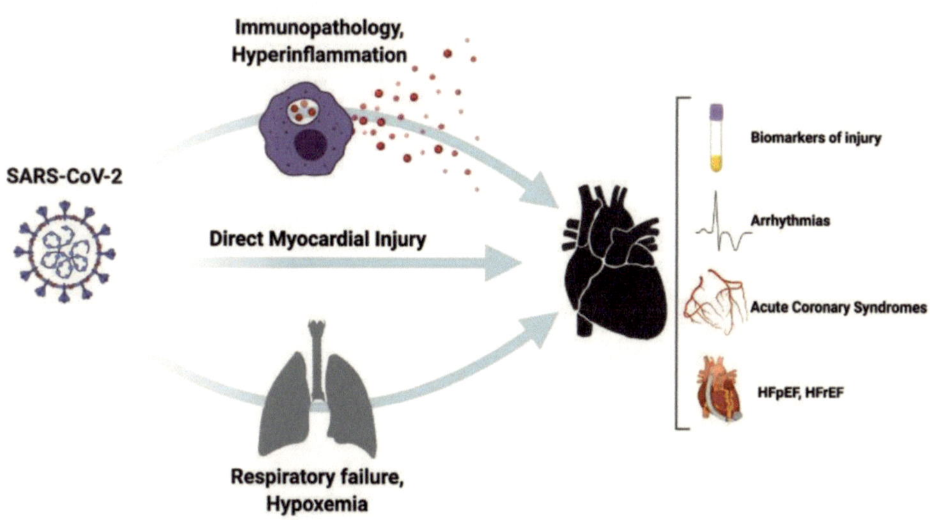

Figure 2.
Mechanisms of cardiac Injury of COVID-19 with clinical sequelae.

tachyarrhythmia attributable to endogenous or exogenous adrenergic stimulation. Systemic infections such as pneumonia have a profound effect on the cardiovascular system, including an increase in oxygen consumption and coronary plaque vulnerability. Myocardial involvement caused by cytokine storm or cardiomyocyte apoptosis triggered by excessive intracellular calcium in response to tissue hypoxia constitutes the indirect response of COVID-19 [4]. Myocardial ischemia occurs in the setting of shock, prolonged tachycardia, or severe respiratory failure, known as type 2 acute myocardial injury (AMI) or acute atherothrombosis, known as type 1 AMI. Type 1 myocardial infarction occurs in the setting of atherothrombosis, which may be triggered by a proinflammatory and prothrombotic state. Type 2 myocardial infarction is most likely in patients with prolonged oxygen supply or demand imbalance with hypoxia, hypotension, or tachycardia. Finally, both myocarditis and takotsubo syndrome have been reported in patients with confirmed COVID-19 and in those without COVID-19 who had experienced severe anxiety due to the pandemic or with concomitant infections.

4. Cardiac troponin and high sensitivity troponin

Cardiac troponin (cTn) is a well-studied and commonly used marker of cardiovascular disease. Troponin is a calcium-regulatory protein for the calcium regulation of contractile function in skeletal and cardiac muscles. Troponin is a complex of three different subunits, troponins C, I, and T, which share characteristic functions of troponin, such as the binding of Ca^{2+} (troponin C), the inhibition of actomyosin interaction (troponin I), and the binding to tropomyosin (troponin T). Troponin is nearly undetectable in unaffected muscle, but troponin levels rise several hours after the onset of myocardial injury. Elevated levels of troponin have been used as a widely accepted marker of cardiac injury. It is detectable up to 10 days after the onset of injury. The degree of elevation of troponin also gives prognostic information on the subsequent outcome as seen in **Figure 3**. Cardiac troponin I levels of 1.0 μg/L or higher or cardiac troponin T levels of 0.1 μg/L or higher are considered elevated. Circulating cTn is a marker of myocardial injury, including

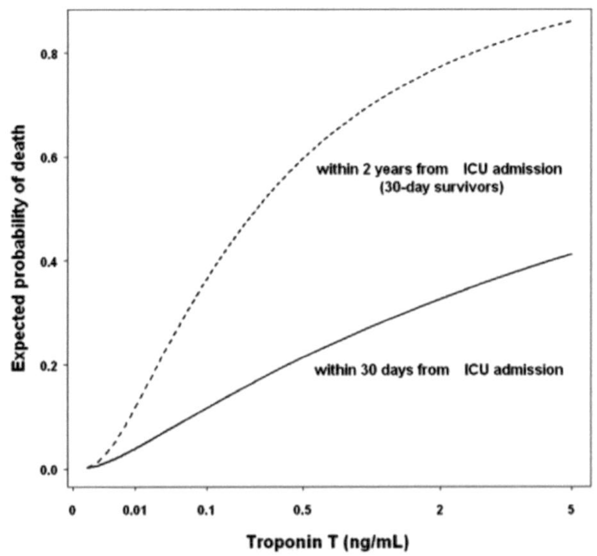

Figure 3.
Relationship of troponin T and expected probability of death.

but not limited to myocardial infarction or myocarditis. There has been growing evidence of higher mortality rates among patients among those patients with underlying cardiovascular disease. The values of cardiac troponin and its elevations above normal concentrations in a patient with COVID-19 should be seen as the combination of the presence or extent of pre-existing cardiac disease and the acute myocardial injury related to COVID-19 and its complications. It further acts as a quantitative marker of this injury. It has been proposed that there are three phases of troponin elevation: first, when cardiac troponin increases mostly reflect ongoing comorbidities, commonly seen at the time of are admission; second, with a critical illness like ARDS; third, specific COVID-19 complications such as pulmonary embolism, stroke, endothelitis and myocarditis. Patients with COVID-19 admitted to the hospital, at 30-day follow up with higher cTn (concentrations greater than ≥21 ng/L) have been associated independently with a higher risk of all-cause mortality. Cardiac troponin elevations, even in small amounts (≥21 ng/L) provide a better prediction of 30-day all-cause mortally and severe course of the disease than other commonly used biomarkers for inflammation including C-reactive protein (CRP), lactate dehydrogenase (LDH), and D-dimer. Furthermore, greater elevations (cTn > 90 ng/L) correlate with higher risk of death than small concentrations (cTn > 30–90 ng/L). Patients with cTn concentrations in the third centile had about six times the all-cause mortality as well as cardiovascular mortality as compared to patients in the first tertile. Higher troponin concentrations are also related to a higher risk of death within 30 days as well as 2 years. Concentrations remained in the normal range in the majority of survivors. High sensitivity troponin I (hs-TnI) is a newer, more sensitive marker of disease progression and mortality in patients with cardiac disease [5]. It was established to be a better marker than those used to determine generalized inflammation including D-dimer and lymphocyte count. Raised hc-TnI in patients admitted with COVID-19 has also been showed to correlate with increased requirements of invasive as well as non-invasive ventilation, development of acute respiratory distress syndrome (ARDS) as well as acute kidney injury (AKI). Studies revealed that the elevated hs-TnI levels were closely correlated with the prognosis and mortality risk of COVID-19 patients. Specifically, the mortality risk increased by 20.8% when the hs-TnI level increased by 1 unit in one such study. However, it is noteworthy to remember that elevated levels are common in hospitalized patients, and are most commonly in the setting of type 2 myocardial infarction (myocardial oxygen supply-demand imbalance) or non-ischemic causes of myocardial injury. Marked elevations of cardiac troponin in patients without critical illnesses such as ARDS, may indicate the presence of takotsubo syndrome, myocarditis, or type 1 AMI triggered by COVID-19. In the absence of symptoms or electrocardiographic changes suggestive of type 1 acute myocardial injury, imaging studies including echocardiography and/cardiac magnetic resonance should be considered to detect left ventricular systolic dysfunction as a new and treatable condition. Patients with symptoms suggestive of type 1 AMI should be treated according to European Society of Cardiology (ESC) guidelines irrespective of COVID-19 diagnosis or suspicion. These patients should undergo rapid coronary angiography under specific catheter personnel. Patients with COVID-19 or other pneumonia who are critically ill with septic shock or ARDS, even marked cardiac troponin elevations are much more likely the consequence of critical illness. The recognition of myocardial injury with elevated cardiac troponin and hs-TnI, given its sensitivity as an early and precise marker of end-organ dysfunction, can prompt timely triage to a critical care unit and informs the measures to improve tissue oxygenation and perfusion with the use of inotropes and vasopressors. Further research is required to elucidate the value of cardiac troponin and high sensitivity troponin I in COVID-19.

5. Creatinine kinase

Creatine Kinase (CK) is an intracellular enzyme present primarily in skeletal muscle, myocardium, and brain. Disruption of cell membranes due to hypoxia or other injury releases CK from cytosol to systemic circulation. CK is a dimeric molecule composed of 2 subunits, namely M and B. Combinations of these subunits form the isoenzymes CK-MM, CK-MB, and CK-BB. A significant concentration of CK-MB isoenzyme is found almost exclusively in the myocardium, and therefore elevations in CK-MB levels in serum is highly specific and sensitive for myocardial injury. Normal reference values for CK-MB range from 3 to 5% of total CK, or 5 to 25 IU/L. Creatine Kinase as a marker of myocardial injury has been largely replaced by troponin in clinical practice. As with troponins, several mechanisms explain the elevated cardiac markers in severe COVID-19: viral myocarditis, cytokine-driven myocardial damage, microangiopathy, and unmasked CAD. Myocardial ACE2 receptors are targets for SARS-CoV-2. A hypothesis is that SARS-CoV-2 induces indirect cardiovascular injury through activation of the immune system. The virus attaches to the pattern recognition receptors (PRRs), that initiate host-immune defense. This host-immune defense system, in turn, induces inflammatory reactance that culminates in a cytokine storm. The cytokine storm is caused by the release of reactive oxygen species (ROS), endogenous nitric oxide (NO), and damage-associated molecular proteins (DAMPs) by the injured myocardium that ultimately leads to myocardial injury. Cytokines and host-immune dysregulation cause direct and indirect cardiac injury, leading to an increase in troponin and CK-MB. A meta-analysis showed that when compared with mortality, COVID-19 patients who died had significantly higher biomarkers, including CK-MB. Another meta-analysis showed that there was a significantly higher CK level in patients who died compared to patients who survived, whereas the patients who were critically ill did not have significantly higher CK levels compared to the patients who were not critically ill.

6. Natriuretic peptides

Natriuretic peptides represent a change of intracardial pressure, especially atrial pressure, and thus is also used as an important cardiac function indicator. These include Brain-type natriuretic peptide (BNP), NT-proBNP, and mid-regional pro atrial natriuretic peptide. Nartiuretic peptides are trigger by hemodynamic stress and heart failure, intracardiac filling pressures, end diastolic wall stress, and hypoxemia. In patients who are not critically ill, BNP/pro-BNP elevations have a high positive predictive value for heart failure. However, in patients who are critically ill, the elevations are likely in the presence of hemodynamic stress and heart failure. Several studies have identified heart failure as a significant manifestation of COVID-19. Heart failure in COVID-19 patients is postulated to occur as a result of the severe immune system reaction and cytokine storm [6, 7]. The virus down-regulates the angiotensin-converting enzyme 2 (ACE2), leading to increased levels of angiotensin II. Further, this causes increased inflammation, thrombosis, and hypertension. Abnormalities NT-proBNP, were associated with higher in-hospital mortality in all patients and in severe patients. Studies were done to estimate the cumulative in-hospital mortality among patients severe COVID-19 patients. The mortality rates were the highest with elevated hs-cTnI and NT-proBNP, followed by elevated NT-proBNP and normal hs-cTnI, elevated hs-cTnI and normal NT-proBNP, and normal hs-cTnI and NT-proBNP. The combination of these two cardiac markers together was found to be more valuable than cardiac troponin alone in determining the prognosis of COVID-19 patients. There has been one retrospective study that reported a correlation between first and peak BNP values to predict the need for mechanical ventilation and mortality respectively. Pro-BNP levels elevated above 167.5 pg./mL are associated with an increased risk of mortality in patients receiving mechanical ventilation. Furthermore, along with the strong association of mortality in patients admitted to the hospital with COVID-19, the elevation of natriuretic peptides could be used as an early indicator for the presence of left and right ventricular systolic dysfunction independently. Identification of ventricular systolic dysfunction, if a treatable dysregulation, will help in decreased mortality and improved outcomes in patients.

7. Newer biomarkers

7.1 MR-proADM—mid-regional proadrenomedullin

ADM is a multipotent regulatory peptide with several biological activities including vasodilator, positive inotropic, diuretic, natriuretic, and bronchodilator. It is widely expressed throughout the body, including bone, adrenal cortex, kidney, lung, blood vessels, and heart. ADM is even present in pulmonary pneumocytes type 2, smooth muscle cells, neurons, and immune cells. It is upregulated by hypoxia, inflammatory cytokines, bacterial products, and shear stress. As ADM measurement is complicated, mid-regional proadrenomedullin (MR-proADM) is being considered as an estimate of ADM [8–10]. High levels of MR-proADM are reported in septic patients. These have been shown to be particularly specific in prognostic value, not only for early diagnosis in the context of patients initially presenting to the Emergency Department (ED) but also for risk stratification and prognosis in critically ill patients in Intensive Care Units (ICU). A study from Italy in 2020 aimed to describe the utility of MR-proADM as a prognostic biomarker in severe COVID-19 infection. Fifty seven patients who were admitted to the ICU with COVID-19 infection were studied. Multivariate logistic regression models demonstrated that MR-proADM was an independent predictor of mortality [11].

7.2 GDF-15—growth differentiation factor 15

Growth differentiation factor 15 (GDF-15) is a member of the transforming growth factor β superfamily and is widely distributed in low concentrations in most organs [12]. Physiological GDF-15 concentrations increase with age, while the expression is upregulated in pathological states through several pathways that mediate damage to the heart, lungs, liver, and kidneys including inflammation, oxidative stress, and hypoxia. Elevated concentrations of circulating GDF-15 have been identified in multiple disease entities like CVD, sepsis, cancer, and diabetes. GDF-15 levels seem to be a robust predictor of disease progression.

A clinical trial from Norway in 2020 looked at the value of GDF-15 as a biomarker in 123 patients admitted with COVID-19, GDF-15 was elevated in 80% of patients hospitalized with COVID-19, and higher concentrations were associated with SARS-CoV-2 viremia, hypoxemia, and worse clinical outcome. Moreover, GDF15 concentrations were more closely associated with poor outcomes than established biomarkers in COVID-19, including cTnT, NT-proBNP, CRP, and D-dimer. Greater increases in GDF-15 during hospitalization were also independently associated with worse outcomes.

7.3 Cardiac enzymes and prognosis

The prognostic role of cardiac markers in patients hospitalized with COVID-19 is remarkably similar to those in patients with viral pneumonia due to influenza, as well as for pneumonia and ARDS in general in addition to certain unique characteristics. Increased concentrations of cTn, hs-TnI, pro-BNP have been showed to have a correlation with increased mortality and severity of COVID-19 pneumonia [13]. Mild elevations in cardiac troponin concentrations, particularly in older patients with pre-existing cardiac disease, are often explained by the combination of known or unknown pre-existing cardiac disease and acute myocardial injury related to COVID-19 or any pneumonia [14, 15]. It is imperative to be aware of the potential use of anticoagulants and anti-cytokine therapies as conceivable therapeutic options, which need to be further explored in clinical trials. In such cases, when there is evidence of cardiac injury as indicated by elevated troponins, possibilities such as myocardial microthrombi should be considered. In patients with established or suspected COVID-19 normal hs-cTnT/I and BNP/NT-proBNP concentrations, of course always in conjunction with vital parameters including pulse oximetry, can reassure physicians that outpatient management is feasible [16]. These insights can help overcome the limitations in determining the prognosis and stratification of patients as well as predicting their mortality. The cardiovascular system has been shown to be a major contributor to the proportion of deaths classified as "non-cardiovascular" by current classification schemes. An example of this is severe sepsis, mortality rates of which have a high contribution from dysfunction of the cardiac system, determined by the enzymes discussed above. Various other cardiac and vascular biomarkers are being studied in ongoing COVID-19 research. An example of this is the emerging data that growth differentiation factor 15 (GDF-15), a member of the transforming growth factor β superfamily that is released by stress due to change in hemodynamics as well as inflammation has better prognostic accuracy than established biomarkers in patients with COVID-19.

8. Limitations

Cardiac troponin provides incremental prognostic information, only in addition to other routinely available variables. These include vital signs, clinical judgment, and other inflammatory markers such as C-reactive protein and D-dimer. Moreover, the increased implementation of these markers, such as elevated cardiac troponin in routine practice might result in inappropriate diagnostic and therapeutic interventions [17]. For example, some clinicians may elect to perform a coronary angiography in the setting of an isolated cardiac troponin elevation. These elevations would likely be in the setting of supply-demand imbalance, and less likely due to type 1 acute myocardial injury. These increased interventions also serve as a possible cause for increased harm to patients as well as the medical care team due to increased exposure to COVID-19 patients. Even non-invasive investigations may be associated with the harm caused due to the risk associated with unnecessarily transporting critically ill patients through the hospital. Hence, firm indications for testing are advocated for [18]. However, when appropriate indications are present, one should not withhold essential evaluations. There is concern that measuring cardiac troponin during the initial blood sampling in the ED may delay patient disposition, as elevated levels require additional investigation, and possibly consultation. In patients with COVID-19 and patients with ARDS, there is currently no evidence that any intervention triggered by an elevation in cardiac troponin concentration will have an impact on patient outcomes.

9. Conclusion

As we continue to learn about COVID-19 and its cardiac consequences, widespread use of cardiac markers in routine clinical practice will increase large datasets leading to better clinical characterization, cardiac imaging, and follow up leading to a better understanding of the pathophysiological mechanisms leading to cardiomyocyte injury in COVID-19. As blood tests are routinely done on patients hospitalized with COVID-19, cardiac biomarkers are easy, cost-effective and accessible method of screening for cardiac complications of COVID-19 and determining the overall prognosis of COVID-19 patients.

10. Summary

- In patients with COVID-19 presenting with chest discomfort or dyspnea, cardiac troponin, myoglobin, natriuretic peptides, help physicians in the initial assessment.

- Small increases in cardiac troponin concentrations are frequently seen and have multiple causes including myocardial oxygen supply-demand mismatch, myocarditis, and a systemic inflammatory response syndrome.

- Compared with other biomarkers, elevated peak troponin I had the greatest predictive value for mortality associated with COVID-19.

- If there is clear evidence of myocardial ischemia considering all available evidence, patients should be managed as acute coronary syndromes.

- Cardiac troponin, creatinine kinase, and natriuretic peptide are indicated as valuable tests in patients with worsening COVID-19.

Author details

Meher Singha[1], Abhishek Madathanapalli[1] and Raj Parikh[2*]

1 Department of Internal Medicine, University of Connecticut, Farmington, CT, United States

2 Division of Pulmonary and Critical Care Medicine, Hartford Hospital, Hartford, CT, United States

*Address all correspondence to: raj.parikh210@gmail.com

References

[1] Kermali M, Khalsa RK, Pillai K, Ismail Z, Harky A. The role of biomarkers in diagnosis of COVID-19—A systematic review. Life Sciences. 2020;**254**:117788. DOI: 10.1016/j.lfs.2020.117788. Epub 2020 May 13

[2] Mueller C, Giannitsis E, Jaffe AS, Huber K, Mair J, Cullen L, et al. Cardiovascular biomarkers in patients with COVID-19. European Heart Journal Acute Cardiovascular Care. 2021;**10**(3):310-319. DOI: 10.1093/ehjacc/zuab009

[3] Lee PY, Day-Lewis M, Henderson LA, Friedman KG, Lo J, Roberts JE, et al. Distinct clinical and immunological features of SARS-CoV-2-induced multisystem inflammatory syndrome in children. The Journal of Clinical Investigation. 2020;**130**(11):5942-5950. DOI: 10.1172/JCI141113

[4] Guagliumi G, Sonzogni A, Pescetelli I, Pellegrini D, Finn AV. Microthrombi and ST-Segment-elevation myocardial infarction in COVID-19. Circulation. 2020;**142**(8):804-809. DOI: 10.1161/CIRCULATIONAHA.120.049294. Epub 2020 Jul 17

[5] Chapman AR, Bularga A, Mills NL. High-sensitivity cardiac troponin can be an ally in the fight against COVID-19. Circulation. 2020;**141**(22):1733-1735. DOI: 10.1161/CIRCULATIONAHA.120.047008. Epub 2020 Apr 6

[6] Shafi AMA, Shaikh SA, Shirke MM, Iddawela S, Harky A. Cardiac manifestations in COVID-19 patients—A systematic review. Journal of Cardiac Surgery. 2020;**35**(8):1988-2008. DOI: 10.1111/jocs.14808. Epub 2020 Jul 11

[7] Latif F, Farr MA, Clerkin KJ, Habal MV, Takeda K, Naka Y, et al. Characteristics and outcomes of recipients of heart transplant with coronavirus disease 2019. JAMA Cardiology. 2020;**5**(10):1165-1169. DOI: 10.1001/jamacardio.2020.2159

[8] Citgez E, Zuur-Telgen M, van der Palen J, van der Valk P, Stolz D, Brusse-Keizer M. Stable-state midrange proadrenomedullin is associated with severe exacerbations in COPD. Chest. 2018;**154**(1):51-57. DOI: 10.1016/j.chest.2018.02.006

[9] Cheung BM, Tang F. Adrenomedullin: Exciting new horizons. Recent Patents on Endocrine, Metabolic and Immune Drug Discovery. 2012;**6**(1):4-17. DOI: 10.2174/187221412799015263

[10] Krintus M, Kozinski M, Braga F, Kubica J, Sypniewska G, Panteghini M. Plasma midregional proadrenomedullin (MR-proADM) concentrations and their biological determinants in a reference population. Clinical Chemistry and Laboratory Medicine. 2018;**56**(7):1161-1168. DOI: 10.1515/cclm-2017-1044

[11] Montrucchio G, Sales G, Rumbolo F, Palmesino F, Fanelli V, Urbino R, et al. Effectiveness of mid-regional pro-adrenomedullin (MR-proADM) as prognostic marker in COVID-19 critically ill patients: An observational prospective study. PLoS One. 2021;**16**(2):e0246771. DOI: 10.1371/journal.pone.0246771

[12] Schuetz P, Wolbers M, Christ-Crain M, Thomann R, Falconnier C, Widmer I, et al. Prohormones for prediction of adverse medical outcome in community-acquired pneumonia and lower respiratory tract infections. Critical Care. 2010;**14**(3):R106

[13] Peiró ÓM, Carrasquer A, Sánchez-Gimenez R, Lal-Trehan N, Del-Moral-Ronda V, Bonet G, et al. Biomarkers and short-term prognosis in

COVID-19. Biomarkers. 2021;**26**(2): 119-126. DOI: 10.1080/1354750X. 2021.1874052. Epub 2021 Jan 18

[14] Fan H, Zhang L, Huang B, Zhu M, Zhou Y, Zhang H, et al. Cardiac injuries in patients with coronavirus disease 2019: Not to be ignored. International Journal of Infectious Diseases. 2020;**96**:294-297. DOI: 10.1016/j. ijid.2020.05.024. Epub 2020 May 11

[15] He X, Wang L, Wang H, Xie Y, Yu Y, Sun J, et al. Factors associated with acute cardiac injury and their effects on mortality in patients with COVID-19. Scientific Reports. 2020;**10**(1):20452. DOI: 10.1038/s41598-020-77172-1

[16] Manocha KK, Kirzner J, Ying X, Yeo I, Peltzer B, Ang B, et al. Troponin and other biomarker levels and outcomes among patients hospitalized with COVID-19: Derivation and validation of the HA_2T_2 COVID-19 mortality risk score. Journal of the American Heart Association. 2021;**10**(6):e018477. DOI: 10.1161/ JAHA.120.018477. Epub 2020 Oct 30

[17] Wungu CDK, Khaerunnisa S, Putri EAC, Hidayati HB, Qurnianingsih E, Lukitasari L, et al. Meta-analysis of cardiac markers for predictive factors on severity and mortality of COVID-19. International Journal of Infectious Diseases. 2021;**105**:551-559. DOI: 10.1016/j. ijid.2021.03.008. Epub 2021 Mar 9

[18] Akhmerov A, Marbán E. COVID-19 and the heart. Circulation Research. 2020;**126**(10):1443-1455. DOI: 10.1161/ CIRCRESAHA.120.317055. Epub 2020 Apr 7

Chapter 3

A High Fidelity Transmural Anisotropic Ventricular Tissue Model Function to Investigate the Interaction Mechanisms of Drug: An In-Silico Model for Pharmacotherapy

Srinivasan Jayaraman and Ponnuraj Kirthi Priya

Abstract

A high fidelity transmural anisotropic ventricular tissue model consisting of endocardial, mid myocardial, and epicardial myocytes were configured to investigate drug interaction, such as Hydroxychloroquine (HCQ), under hypoxia conditions without and with pro-arrhythmic comorbidity like hypokalemia in (a) ventricular tissue b) its arrhythmogenesis for different dosages and (b) two different pacing sequences (Normal and tachycardiac). In-silico ventricular modeling indicates HCQ has an insignificant effect on hypoxia with and without comorbidities, except in the combination of mild hypoxia with moderate hypokalemia condition and severe hypoxia with mild hypokalemia where it initiated a re-entrant arrhythmia. Secondly, incorporating drug dosage variations indicates the 10 μM HCQ created PVCs for all settings except in severe hypoxia conditions where re-entrant arrhythmia occurred. In addition to the dosage of HCQ utilized for treatment, the pacing protocol also influences the appearance of re-entrant arrhythmia only for severe hypoxia with 10 μM HCQ dosage alone. For all other conditions, including tachycardiac pacing protocol, no arrhythmia occurred. These findings infer that the arrhythmic fatality rate due to HCQ treatment for hypoxia can be effectively alleviated by subtly altering or personalizing the dosage of HCQ and aid in the treatment of hypoxia-induced symptoms caused by COVID.

Keywords: Hydroxychloroquine, Hypoxia, Hypokalemia, Azithromycin, Ventricular Arrhythmia, Transmural Tissue, COVID-19

1. Introduction

Precision medicine is significantly focused and promoted due to the development of next-generation sequencing, which implies high throughput and lower cost. Even though molecular and cell biology has improved basic understanding of many diseases, novel and pandemic diseases like Severe Acute Respiratory Syndrome Coronavirus (SARS-CoV-2) have many unanswered questions on infection mechanism, progression, and impact of symptom-based treatment using "off label" drugs. For instance, Hydroxychloroquine (HCQ), an antimalarial drug widely used to boost the immune system, was attempted or explored towards treating COVID-19. The US Food and Drugs Administration (FDA) and WHO initially approved HCQ as an emergency medicine based on laboratory and clinical studies data. Irrespective of earlier findings suggesting that long-term (over 5 years) intake of HCQ is likely to contribute to the development of retinopathy, include QRS widening, QT interval prolongation, ventricular arrhythmias like Torsades de pointes (TdP), hypokalemia and hypotension [1, 2], in-vitro studies reported the potential activity of HCQ on SARS-CoV-2 [3, 4]. On a positive note, in experiments performed on mouse atria, Capel et al. [5] reported that HCQ acted as a bradycardiac agent (reducing the spontaneous beating rate) in sinoatrial cells via a dose-dependent reduction of multiple ionic currents: 'funny' current (I_f), L-type calcium current (I_{CaL}) and rapid delayed rectifier potassium current (I_{Kr}). Modeling of drug cardiotoxicity at the cellular level focuses predominantly on reducing I_{Kr} current and leads to prolongation of APD in cells and QT interval in whole heart level, thereby leading to arrhythmias like TdP [6]. However, a clinical study in France [7] reported that either HCQ alone or in combination with azithromycin is efficient in treating COVID-19. However, Sarkar et al., 2012 [8] reported that one population of cell differs from another (i.e healthy vs. diseased) and electrophysiological variability manifests at each level, from molecular, cellular, organ, and organism level. Hence, considering the outcome of previous clinical evidence of HCQ on normal cells may be inadequate to provide the exact impact of the effect of HCQ on virus infected cells or tissue. As our particular interest is in the human cardiac system; specifically electrophysiology, we wish to emphasis the variability of COVID-19 in cardiac system. Clinical observations reported by Mercuro et al. [9] shows the median baseline QT_c was 455 ms in 90 COVID-19 patients and in presence of HCQ, it increased to 473 ms. Among those who received HCQ alone, 19% had QT_c prolongation of 500 ms or more, 13% had a change in QT_c of 60 ms or more and 1 case of Torsade de Pointes (TdP) was reported. Thus it's very evident that investigating and understanding the cardiac manifestation mechanism due to medication like HCQ drug is critical.

Li X et al.'s study in 2019 on 175 patients with COVID-19 reported that, 39 patients had severe hypokalemia (under 3 mmol/L), 69 had moderate hypokalemia (3–3.5 mmol/L) and 67 were normokalemia (over 3.5 mmol/L) [10]. He et al., [11] proposed that ACE-2 signaling pathways may play a role in cardiac injury while hypoxemia caused by COVID-19 may cause damage to myocardial cells. Severe hypoxemia occurring in lungs of COVID-19 patients has been linked to loss of lung perfusion regulation and hypoxic vasoconstriction [12]. Acute viral infections like that of COVID-19 have been known to cause type 1 or 2 myocardial infarction though the frequency of STE in these patients is unclear [13]. All these resulted in the liberal use of HCQ globally, in spite of contempt of paucity of evidence and adverse effect [3] for a short span of time.

During this situation, Wang et al. reported that treating COVID-19 with a combination of HCQ and AZM elicited electrical alternates, re-entrant circuits and the wave breaks [14]. Further, this clinical study reported that different dosages of HCQ blocked the various ionic currents: I_{Na}, I_{CaL}, I_{Kr} and I_{K1} with different intensity. Based on the [15] finding, HCQ treatment for COVID-19 lead to ventricular arrhythmia and death in hospitalized COVID patients, In May 2020, WHO suspended the emergency usage of HCQ; later, this study article was retracted due to reporting of fabricated data. There is no clinical evidence that provides the detailed mechanism of HCQ's safety or adversity, particularly the cardiac cell and tissue, i.e., under what scenarios the target drug interaction may cause arrhythmias in patients.

Although various researchers have attempted to study the pharmacokinetics of HCQ: it's the inhibitory mechanism on human cells under normal conditions and various abnormal pathologies, for the reasons noted, it is critical to zero down the effect of a drug and explains its response range. Such comprehensive study, either using in-vivo or clinical studies, is difficult in a short period with present-day technology. In this situation, computational models can help to elucidate and overcome the following aspects:

- The effect of COVID-19 infection on electrophysiological properties of ventricular tissue
- Lack of clinical evidence that provides a detailed influence of HCQ on COVID-19 infected cardiac tissue. For example, changes in ECG, mechanism, and potential severity of ventricular arrhythmias like TdP
- Mechanistic understanding of HCQ on ventricular tissues under comorbid scenarios, such as varying intensities of hypokalemia.

To address the above gaps, we develop a 2D transmural anisotropic ventricular tissue model framework that can help in primarily understanding the COVID-19 effect on the ventricular tissue, including the response to pharmacological agents like HCQ. Two variations of COVID-19; mild and severe infection are explored. Secondly, different levels of hypokalemia (mild, moderate and severe) along with COVID-19 are introduced one at a time to understand its effect on ventricular tissue In each case, the variations in the QT interval and T-peak are recorded. Finally, the tissue is excited with premature stimuli to analyze under which of the above three conditions the tissue becomes pro- arrhythmic. Although studies have established that HCQ induces QT prolongation, TdP arises only in certain scenarios. This study is an attempt to address the possibilities under which an arrhythmia is generated at the tissue level in presence of the above mentioned conditions.

2. Transmural cardiac tissue model

The 2D transmural section of the ventricular wall, is represented by an array of 250×100 cells, consisting of endocardial (endo), midmydocardial (M) and

Condition	Ionic current	Change
HCQ	I_{Kr}	35% reduction
	I_{CaL}	12% reduction
Hypokalemia1	K_o^+	85% reduction
Hypokalemia2	K_o^+	55% reduction
Hypokalemia3	K_o^+	45% reduction
Mild COVID-19	$[ATP]_i$ $k_{0.5}$	5.5 mM 0.125
Severe COVID-19	$[ATP]_i$	5 mM
	$k_{0.5}$	0.250

Table 1.
Change in parameters for different conditions.

epicardial(epi) cells. The depolarisation and repolarisation patterns generated from the tissue are validated by simulating pseudo ECGs. The action potentials of different types of cardiomyocytes are described by the Ten Tusscher (TP06) model [16]. A stimulus current of amplitude 52 μA is applied for 1 ms is used to excite specific cell. The parameters of the model, tissue characteristics and integration scheme are adopted from Priya et al., 2017 [17]. The change in cardiomyocyte's ionic current parameters in the various configurations: hypokalemia and COVID-19 are summarized in **Table 1**.

As COVID-19 has been linked to causing hypoxemia [11], which in turn leads to hypoxia, this condition was included in the cardiac myocytes by increasing intracellular ATP concentration which would in turn lead to activation of an ATP sensitive potassium current. Using the formulation of Shaw and Rudy [18], ATP activated K^+ current is described by the following formula

$$I_{ATP} = G_{k,ATP} \frac{1}{1 + \left(\frac{[ATP]_i}{k_{0.5}}\right)^H} \left(\frac{[K_o^+]}{5.4}\right)^n (V_m - E_k) \tag{1}$$

where $G_{k,ATP}$ is the maximum conductance of I_{ATP} current and has a value of 3.9 nS/cm^2, H and n have a value of 2 and 0.24 respectively. The intracellular ATP concentration ($[ATP]_i$) under normal condition is 6.8 mM, but it decreases to 5.5 mM in mild hypoxia and 5 mM in severe hypoxia respectively. Similarly, $k_{0.5}$ is 0.042 for normal condition, 0.125 and 0.25 for mild and severe hypoxia respectively [19]. Henceforth, in this study, hypoxia would be referred as COVID-19 condition. Further, reduction in the rapid delayed rectifying potassium current (I_{Kr}) and I_{CaL} by 35% and 12% respectively in atrial cells as reported by [5] is adapted in our model.

To investigate the benefits and adverse effects of HCQ under control, COVID-19 and comorbid hypokalaemia, the ion channel variations corresponding to these conditions were included in the cells of the tissue one at a time, as reported by [10], the extracellular potassium concentration (Ko^+) is reduced by three stages: 85% as hypokalemia1 (mild), 55% as hypokalemia2 (moderate) and 45% as hypokalemia3 (severe). A regular pacing pulse of 800 ms (corresponding to 75 beats per minute) is applied in the tissue, and the corresponding voltage propagation is analyzed. Further, pseudo ECGs are generated for each of the clinical conditions. The variation in ECG, in particular the QT interval and T-wave morphology, both without and with HCQ and in presence of comorbidity is considered for analysis. Furthermore, the tissue is stimulated with premature stimuli in between the normal beats to study which conditions can initiate or sustain an arrhythmia.

3. Cardiac tissue mechanism(s) in control, COVID-19 and hypokalemia conditions, and with HCQ

To understand the spatiotemporal mechanism of the cardiac tissue, the lower leftmost corner (Cells 1:10,1:2) of the transmural tissue is stimulated. As a result of this stimuli, a convex wavefront propagates from the endo to mid and epi layer from the bottom to the top of the tissue. The repolarisation occurs first in the epi and endo layers, and M-cells in the mid layer are the last to repolarise. Normalized pseudo ECGs are synthesized from this tissue. *Mild* and *severe* COVID-19 conditions are introduced in the tissue to study its effect without and with HCQ. Furthermore, a comorbidity like hypokalemia is included to understand its influence on COVID-

19 conditions. Pseudo ECGs are synthesized for each of these conditions and the QT interval and T-peak are tabulated in **Table 2**.

In control conditions, a 0.345 sec QT interval and 0.2265 mV T-peak occurs. While in *mild* COVID-19, the QT interval and T-peak decreases by 5.79% (0.325) sec and 33.33% (0.151 mV) respectively as seen in **Figure 1(i)**. In combination with HCQ, the QT interval slightly increases by 1.45% (0.340 sec) and T-peak rises by 20.08% (0.181 mV) in comparison with no HCQ. However, it does not reach the control values. Under severe COVID-19 conditions, the QT interval is further reduced by 20.29% (0.275 s) and a negative T-wave peak of −0.17 mV is observed along with a QT depression. This negative T-peak might be representative of ischemia in clinical ECG recordings. In contrast, the effect of HCQ in *severe* COVID-19 is negligible with unchanged QT interval and slight increase in T-peak (−0.153 mV). Here,we have considered a pacing interval of 800 msec (i.e HR is 75 beats/min), so the Bazett QT_c interval is 0.363 sec and 0.307 sec in *mild* and*severe* COVID-19 conditions. Anttonen *et al.*, [20] reported that an individual's QT_c interval < 320 msec is a low rate of all-cause mortality, from which we infer that a patient with *severe* hypoxia is thus not at high risk of mortality from cardiac failure or disorder; unless and otherwise in presence of other comorbidities. On adding HCQ, 0.380 sec

Condition	QT interval (s)	T-peak (mV)
Control	0.345	0.2265
Mild COVID-19	0.325	0.152
Severe COVID-19	0.275	−0.170
Mild COVID-19 with HCQ	0.340	0.181
Severe COVID-19 with HCQ	0.275	−0.153
Hypokalemia1	0.355	0.229
Hypokalemia1 with HCQ	0.375	0.265
Hypokalemia2	0.380	0.217
Hypokalemia2 with HCQ	0.410	0.255
Hypokalemia3	0.390	0.210
Hypokalemia3 with HCQ	0.425	0.246
Hypokalemia1a and Mild COVID-19	0.335	0.127, 0.153
Hypokalemia1 and Mild COVID-19 with HCQ	0.350	0.186
Hypokalemia1 and Severe COVID-19	0.285	−0.16, −0.087
Hypokalemia1 and Severe COVID-19 with HCQ	0.285	−0.14
Hypokalemia2 and Mild COVID-19	0.355	0.141
Hypokalemia2 and Mild COVID-19 with HCQ	0.38	0.174
Hypokalemia2 and Severe COVID-19	0.300	−0.156
Hypokalemia2 and Severe COVID-19 with HCQ	0.305	−0.126
Hypokalemia3 and Mild COVID-19	0.365	0.133
Hypokalemia3 and Mild COVID-19 with HCQ	0.395	0.168
Hypokalemia3 and Severe COVID-19	0.31	−0.155
Hypokalemia3 and Severe COVID-19 with HCQ	0.32	−0.121

Table 2.
Pseudo ECG parameters: T-peak and QT interval duration as a metric for assessing the effect of COVID-19, other comorbidity and in presence of HCQ.

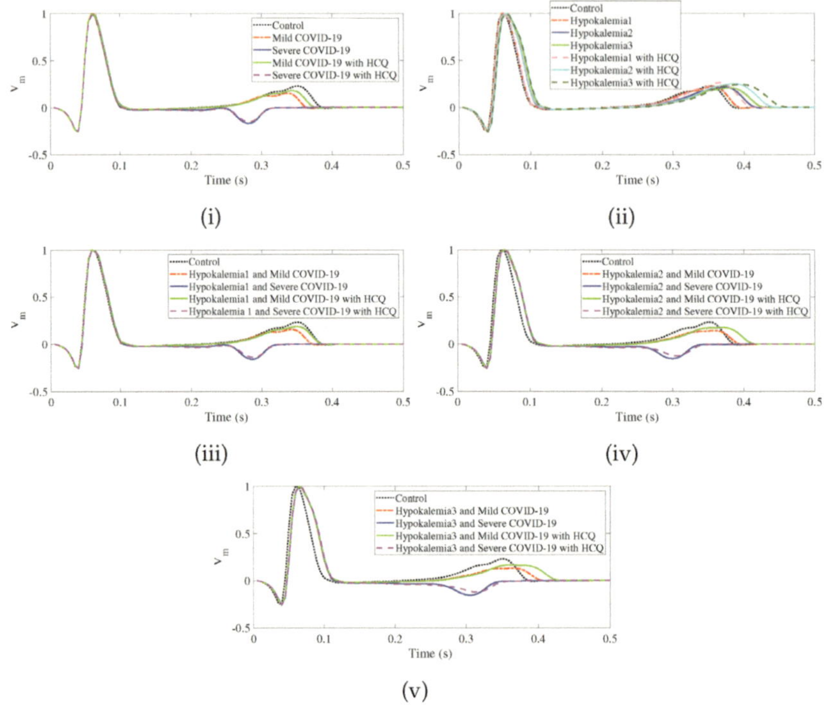

Figure 1.
Pseudo ECGs generated in control and in presence of HCQ under (i)mild and severe COVID-19 (ii) Hypokalemia, (iii)Hypokalemia1 and COVID-19, (iv)Hypokalemia2 and COVID-19 and (v) Hypokalemia3 and COVID-19.

QT_c interval increased in *mild*, while it remains the same in *severe* hypoxia conditions. Mercuro et al. [9] reported that in 90 COVID-19 patients, the median baseline QT_c was 455 (430–474) ms in control vs. 473 [454–487] ms in HCQ conditions. The QT_c values reported in our study are lower than those observed clinically due to the limitation of considering only a segment of the ventricle. However, the percentage increase in APD between control and HCQ in the clinical study of Mercuro et al. is 3.95%. An increase of 4.68% QT_c is observed, on comparing the *mild* COVID-19 and on HCQ inclusion.

Figure 1(ii-v) shows the pseudo ECGs generated for the different combinations of Hypokalemia and COVID-19 as well as in presence of HCQ. In comorbid hypokalemia1 condition as seen in **Figure 1**(ii), the QT interval increases by 2.89% (0.355 s), while the peak amplitude of T-wave increases only by 1.10% (0.229 mV), almost similar to control condition. When exposed to HCQ, the QT interval increases by 8.69% (0.375 ms) and T-peak amplitude increases by 16.99% (0.265 mV) in comparison to control. But, when infected by mild COVID-19, the QT interval decreases by 2.89% (0.335 s), yet a notched T-wave appears with the first T-peak of 0.127 mV and second peak of 0.153 mV is observed. On adding HCQ, the notched T-wave are replaced by positive T-waves. The QT interval is increased by 1.45% (0.350 mV) and T-peak is reduced by 17.88% (0.186 mV) in comparison with control. In contrast to control condition, pre-existing hypokalemia1 with severe COVID-19 reduces the QT interval by 17.39% (0.285 s) and a negative T-peak of 0.16 mV is observed i.e. suggestive of ischemia as seen in **Figure 1**(iii). HCQ drug does not have any noteworthy effect other than slight reduction of T-peak to −0.14 mV.

In hypokalemia2 in **Figure 1**(iv), the QT interval is prolonged by 10.14% (0.380 ms) but T-peak reduced by 4.19% (0.217 mV) is observed, and HCQ exposure increases 18.84% (0.410 ms) QT interval with 12.58% (0.255 mV) increase in T-peak. On considering hypokalemia2 and *mild* COVID-19, the QT interval increases by 2.89% (0.355 s) while T-peak reduces by 37.74% (0.141 mV) in comparison to control, and HCQ inclusion, prolonged QT interval by 10.14% (0.380 s), but reduce the T-peak by 23.17% (0.174 mV). Similar to the hypokalemia1 and COVID-19 scenario, the hypokalemia2 and *severe* COVID-19 we observed, a negative T-peak (0.156 mV) with 13.04% (0.300 s) QT interval reduction. Here too, HCQ has no significant effect, other than a slight increase in the QT interval (0.305 s) and T-peak (0.126 mV).

Finally, in hypokalemia3, **Figure 1(v)**, the QT interval is prolonged by 13.04% (0.390 ms) while the T-peak is reduced by 7.28% (0.210 mV), similar to hypokalemia2 observation. In HCQ presence, the QT interval increases by 23.18% (0.425 ms) and the T-peak increases by 8.61% (0.246 mV) comparing to control. *Mild* COVID-19 has the effect of increasing the QT interval by 5.79% (0.365 s) and reducing the T-peak by 41.28% (0.133 mV). HCQ treatment further prolongs the QT interval by 14.49% (0.395 s) and reduces T-peak by 25.82% (0.168 mV). Similarly for *severe* COVID-19 with hypokalemia3, a negative T-peak of −0.155 mV with 10.14% QT interval reduction (0.310 s) is observed, and on adding HCQ, the QT interval increases to 0.320 s and the T-peak becomes slightly less negative at 0.121 mV. Thus, it can be summarized that irrespective preexisting hypokalemic's severity level, severe COVID-19 can proliferate the risk factor due inverted T-wave presence, that implies the ischemia occurrence.

3.1 Arrhythmogenesis effect of HCQ on COVID-19 infected tissue including and excluding hypokalemia

3.1.1 Premature pacing sequence protocol

The scientific community has well accepted that early or late repolarization of the ventricular myocytes manifest due to ionic imbalances and are regulated by different mechanisms; which are involved in or responsible for various life-threatening cardiac diseases. Further, to understand the arrhythmia mechanism, cardiac tissue is paced with premature beats (PBs) in between the normal pacing beats of 800 ms. Three consecutive PBs (single or two PBs are not effective in creating an arrhythmia) are applied to strive in initiating an arrhythmic pattern. PBs duration is determined as the period the endo cell comes out of the refractory state and are re-excitable. The subsequent sections describe the possibility of occurrence of arrhythmia on pacing the tissue with PBs in *mild* and *severe* COVID-19 configurations, comorbid hypokalemia and on inclusion of HCQ.

3.1.2 Arrhythmogenesis response for mild and severe COVID-19 cardiac tissue: when treated with HCQ

Figure 2 shows the pseudo-ECG on including *mild* and *severe* COVID-19 conditions and on HCQ exposure to cardiac tissue. Under *mild* COVID-19, three PBs of each 295 msec duration are applied after the first beat. The cardiac tissue's mid cells are in a repolarising state when the first PB is applied. This causes the depolarisation from the first PB to travel upward along the endo layer and later depolarise the mid and epi layer, which results in a negative T-wave (**Figure 2(i)**). The depolarisation wavefront from the second PB is not able to excite the cells in the epi layer as they are in a refractory state and this appears as a STE. Further, when the third PB occurs, an inverted T-wave is created as the mid and epi cells depolarize simultaneously. Later in both cases, normal pacing pulses resumed at 1.6 sec and HCQ

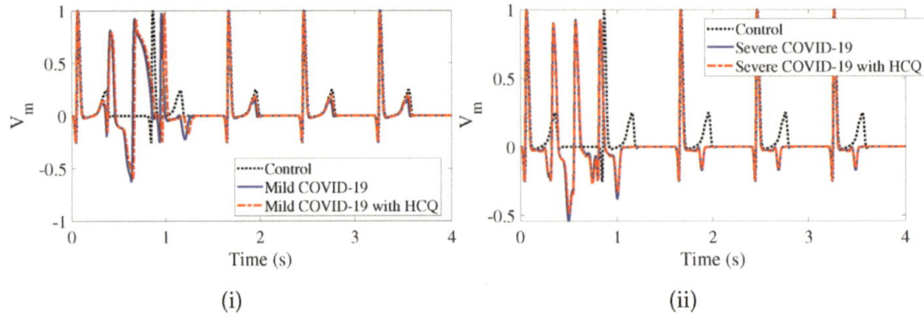

Figure 2.
Pseudo ECG for i)mild COVID-19 and HCQ ii)severe COVID-19 and HCQ.

presence shows a similar trend. This finding is in line with Wang et al. [14] study, where a 10 μM HCQ dosage prolonged the cells APD but did not induce an arrhythmia on decreasing the pacing interval.

In *severe* COVID-19, the three PBs are applied for every 250 msec, that leads to increase in the negative T-peak amplitude, due to the changes in depolarisation and repolarisation pattern; similar to the first PB in mild COVID-19 case. The first and third PBs increases the amplitude of negative T-peak compared to the second PB. The normal ECGs are resumed at 1.6 sec in both scenarios. Results infers that an inverted T-wave morphology (representative of ischemia) can be used as a biomarker for *severe* COVID-19 conditions. Further, HCQ drug causes negligible modifications in the voltage propagation patterns and no effect has been observed in the ECG compared with control.

3.1.3 Arrhythmogenesis mechanism for the pre-existing Hypokalemia of COVID-19 cardiac tissue: when treated with HCQ

To investigate the impact of COVID-19, pseudo ECGs a shown in **Figure 3** are generated on pacing the tissue with PBs in the presence of different degree of Hypokalemia, severity of COVID-19 and on including HCQ.

Hypokalemia1 Infected with COVID-19, with and without HCQ: The tissue is regularly paced every 800 msec. After the first pacing pulse, three premature beats each of 305 msec duration are applied at the same pacing site as indicated in **Figure 3(i)**. It is observed that in the case of hypokalemia1, reentrant activity is generated from 0.37 sec to 1.39 sec and normal beats are resumed from 1.6 sec. On including HCQ and applying three PBs at 325 msec duration each, reentrant activity is generated from 0.38 sec to 2.2 sec and it resumes to normal from 2.4 sec. Hence, there is a 43.96% risk in the arrhythmic activity.

In **Figure 3**(ii), hypokalemia1 and *mild* COVID-19 conditions are included in the tissue, three PBs each of 295 msec are applied after the first beat. The regular pacing interval is 800 msec. When the tissue is excited due to the first PB, the cells in top of endo layer and those in mid and epi layers are in repolarising state. Thus, the wavefront from first PB travels upwards along the endo layer and propagates into the mid and epi layer. When the second PB occurs at 0.59 sec, the mid and epi cells are in repolarising state, thus the wavefront propagates along the endo layer and then enters into the mid and epi layer from the bottom once they come out of refractory state. A similar excitation pattern is observed after the third PB is applied. These changes in depolarisation and repolarisation appears as an arrhythmic-like activity from 0.355 sec to 1.24 sec in the pseudo ECG and normal beats are resumed from 1.6 s. Therefore, it is to be noted that the reentrant activity is not generated. On including HCQ at 305 msec duration of three premature beats,

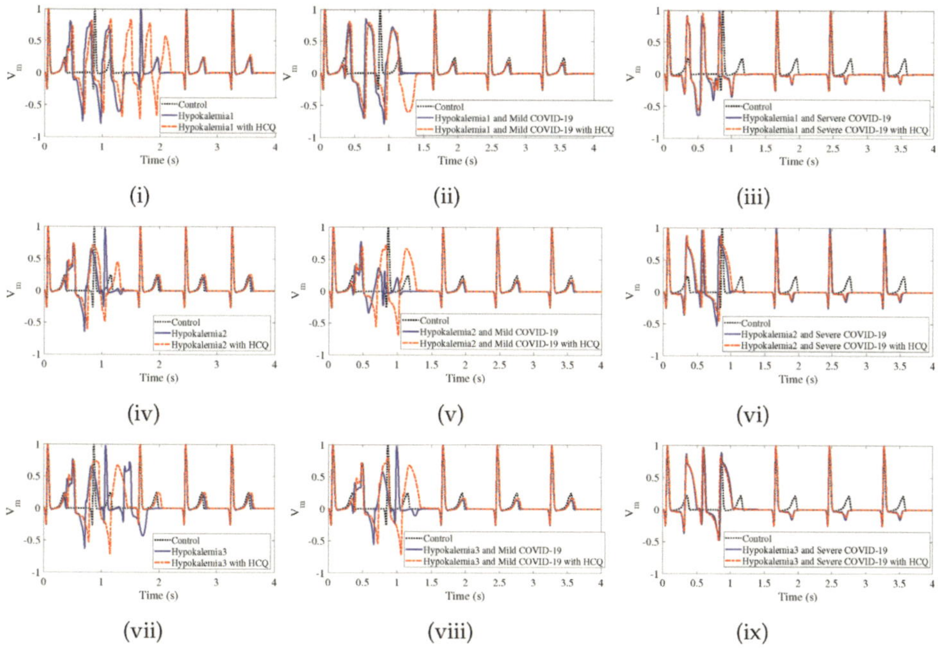

Figure 3.
Pseudo ECG for i)Hypokalemia1 and treated with HCQ, ii)Hypokalemia1 with mild COVID-19 and treated with HCQ iii)Hypokalemia1 with severe COVID-19 and treated with HCQ ii) iv)Hypokalemia2 and treated with HCQ with HCQ, v)Hypokalemia2 with mild COVID-19 and treated with HCQ vi)Hypokalemia2 with severe COVID-19 and treated with HCQ, vii)Hypokalemia3 and treated with HCQ, viii)Hypokalemia3 with mild COVID-19 and treated with HCQ ix)Hypokalemia3 with severe COVID-19 and treated with HCQ.

a similar type of waveform is generated from 0.365 sec to 1.395 sec and normal beats are resumed from 2.4 sec. On the other hand, hypokalemia1 infected with *severe* COVID-19, the absence of HCQ creates a reentrant pattern from 0.315 s to 1.045 s on pacing the tissue with 3 PBs each of 250 ms duration as seen in **Figure 3**(iii). On including HCQ and applying the same pacing protocol, reentry is not generated in the tissue. However, the excitation by the PB creates a similar appearance of ECG waveform. This difference can be seen in **Figure 3**(iii). This shows that HCQ plays a vital role in pre-exisitng hypokalemia1 with COVID-19 cases.

Hypokalemia2 Infected with mild COVID-19, with and without HCQ: Applying three PBs each of 330 msec duration in between the normal pacing pulses in presence of hypokalemia2 does not generate any re-entrant activity as seen in **Figure 3**(iv). The third PB at 0.99 sec generates a negative T-peak of 0.056 mV and the normal activity is resumed from 1.6 sec. However, in presence of HCQ with 355 msec PBs, reentrant activity is generated from 0.4 sec to 1.34 sec and the regular pacing sequence is resumed at 1.6 sec.

Hypokalemia2 and *mild* COVID-19 conditions are included in the tissue and paced with PBs as shown in **Figure 3(v)**. Reentrant activity is observed in the pseudo ECG after pacing with three PBs each of 300 msec duration from 0.355 sec to 0.935 sec. In order to understand the detailed arrhythmogenesis mechanism in hypokalemia2 with *mild* COVID-19 conditions, voltage maps of cardiac tissue are shown in **Figure 4** starting from the application of the first PB at 0.300 sec. At this time, the endo cells at the top and the M-cells and epi cells are still in repolaring state. The depolarisation wave created from this first PB is shown in **Figure 4(a)** at 0.31 sec. This wave proceeds upwards along the endo layer by which time the M-cells are returning to rest state as seen in **Figure 4(b)**. The wavefront then travels along the entire length of endo layer and reenters the mid and epi layers as seen in

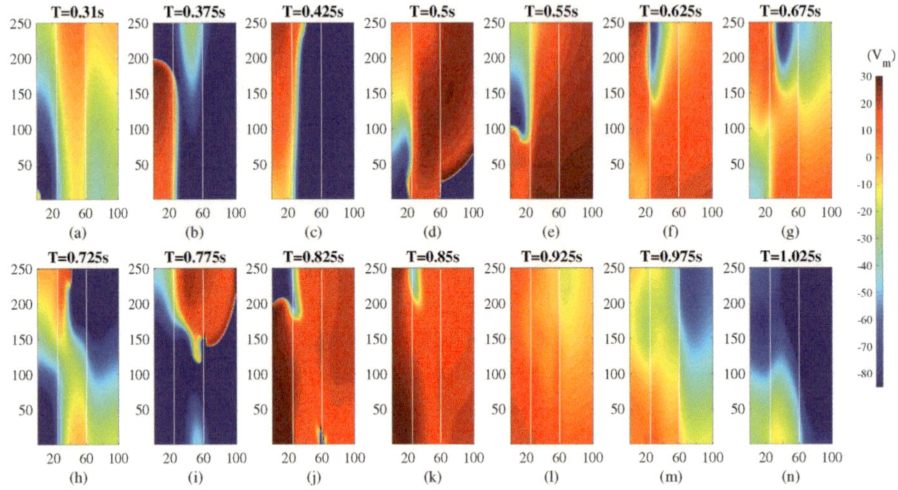

Figure 4.
Voltage maps on applying PBs in Hypokalemia2 with mild COVID-19.

Figure 4(c) and **(d)**. This wavefront then reenters into the endo layer at the bottom of the tissue and travels upwards along the endo layer as seen in **Figure 4(e)** and **(f)**. The second PB is applied at 0.6 sec and during this time the endo cells are already depolarised. This wavefront re-enters into the mid and epi layers by which time the mid and epi cells have repolarised as seen in **Figure 4(g)–(i)**. The wavefront depolarises cells in mid and epi layers and reenters endo layer as seen in **Figure 4(j)–(k)**. The third PB is applied at 0.9 sec and the cells at the pacing site are already depolarised. The cells start repolarising from the epi, mid and endo with cells at the bottom of the endo and mid layer repolarising last as seen in **Figure 4**(ii)(l)–(n). All the cells finally repolarise at 1.085 sec.

On adding HCQ and pacing the tissue with 3 PBs, each of 330 msec duration, in between the regular pacing interval of 800 msec, although arrhythmic-like activity is observed from 0.37 sec to 1.295 sec in the pseudo ECG, this is due to the depolarisation and repolarisation sequence of the cells in the tissue and not because of reentry. Normal beats are resumed from 1.6 sec.

In case of *severe* COVID-19 conditions, the application of three PBs each of 250 msec, gives rise to the pseudo ECG shown in **Figure 3**(vi). The excitation of the first and third PB appear representative of an STE. On introducing HCQ, a similar ECG waveform is observed and no reentry of wavefront is observed.

Hypokalemia3 Infected with COVID-19, with and without HCQ: Similarly, in case of hypokalemia3, reentrant activity is not generated when pacing the tissue with 335 msec duration PBs as seen in **Figure 3**(vii). Inclusion of HCQ causes reentrant activity to appear from 0.415 sec to 1.45 sec on pacing with PBs of 355 msec duration. The regular pacing sequence is resumed at 1.6 sec. Even though HCQ drug is not intended for hypokalemia treatment, here we attempted to understand the role of HCQ in hypokalemia. Result infers that the presence of HCQ is pro-arrhythmic under all severity levels of hypokalemic and would have to be used with caution in such scenarios.

Figure 3(viii) shows the pseudo ECG on including Hypokalemia3 and *mild* COVID-19 conditions in the tissue and pacing with PBs. No reentrant activity is observed even after pacing with three PBs each of 310 msec duration. Similarly, on adding HCQ and pacing the tissue with 3 PBs, each of 330 msec duration, in between the regular pacing interval of 800 ms, no reentrant activity is generated. Normal beats are resumed from 1.6 sec. Under hypokalemia3 and *severe* COVID-19 conditions, the application of three PBs each of 265 ms, gives rise to the pseudo ECG shown in **Figure 3**(ix). Similar to earlier case of hypokalemia2 and severe COVID-19, the excitation of the first and third PB appear representative of an ST-elevation as the epi cells are not depolarised.

4. Dosage effects in COVID-19 infected cardiac tissue: HCQ and with AZM

To understand the influence of different dosages of HCQ alone and in combination with AZM in the COVID-19 infected cardiac tissue, the cardiomyocyte's ionic current parameters are varied based on the clinical study reported by Wang et al., [21], and listed in **Table 3**. To the best of the author's knowledge, prior art studies have not considered the role of temperature (fever) arising due to COVID-19; in this study, we configure the computational model of the ventricular tissue with an elevated temperature of 313.15 Kelvin.

The ECG parameters, namely QT interval, T-peak and QRS duration are extracted from the pseudo ECG and tabulated in **Table 4**. Here, the cardiac tissue is paced with three consecutive premature beats (PBs) with a regular pacing interval of 800 ms (75 bpm). Initialization of the first PB in each case is determined as the endo cell's period comes out of the refractory state and re-excitable. The consecutive beats get reduced by 10 msec. We further extended it in the presence of PBs in *mild* and *severe* COVID-19 to determine the arrhythmia occurrence for various HCQ dosages and with AZM.

In the control ventricular condition, the QT interval is observed to be 0.350 sec, T-peak is 0.232 mV and the QRS duration is 0.07 sec. In the case of adding 1 μM, 10 μM, and 100 μM HCQ, the QT interval increases by 1.42%, 11.43%, and 44.28%, respectively, as shown in **Figure 1(i)**. However, the T-peak decreases by 10.35% and 0.85% under 1 μM and 100 μM HCQ, but, in 10 μM, it increases by 18.10%. Also, QRS duration increased by 7.14% in both 1 μM and 10 μM HCQ and by 21.4% in 100 μM HCQ. Application of PBs in the 1 μM HCQ or 10 μM HCQ configuration, it gives rise to premature ventricular complexes (PVCs), as seen in **Figure 1**(ii) and the regular pacing sequence resumes at 2.4 sec. The appearance of PVC is due to the change in the repolarisation sequence with endo and mid cells repolarising first, followed by the epi cells. For the 100 μM HCQ config, the three PBs gives rise to

Current	**HCQ (1 μM)**	**HCQ (10 μM)**	**HCQ (100 μM)**
I_{Na}	22%	35%	55%
I_{CaL}	12%	12%	40%
I_{Kr}	18%	55%	85%
I_{K1}	10%	20%	80%
	HCQ (1 μM) and AZM	HCQ (10 μM) and AZM	HCQ (100 μM) and AZM
I_{Na}	18%	22%	38%
I_{CaL}	10%	15%	30%
I_{Kr}	30%	62%	90%
I_{Ks}	18%	20%	22%
I_{K1}	10%	30%	82%

Table 3.
Ionic currents for different dosages of HCQ and with AZM represented by in-vitro study [21].

Dosage (μM)	Medication	Disease Condition	QT interval (sec)	T peak (mV)	QRS duration (sec)
	No Medication	Control	0.350	0.232	0.070
		Mild COVID	0.325	0.152	0.070
		severe COVID	0.275	−0.170	0.070
1	HCQ	Control	0.355	0.208	0.075
1	HCQ	*Mild* COVID	0.330	0.110, 0.124	0.075
1	HCQ	*severe* COVID	0.265	−0.206	0.070
1	HCQ with AZM	Control	0.375	0.24	0.070
1	HCQ with AZM	*Mild* COVID	0.350	0.151	0.070
1	HCQ with AZM	*severe* COVID	0.285	−0.194	0.065
10	HCQ	Control	0.390	0.274	0.075
10	HCQ	*Mild* COVID	0.365	0.194	0.075
10	HCQ	*severe* COVID	0.290	−0.137	0.070
10	HCQ with AZM	Control	0.420	0.319	0.070
10	HCQ with AZM	*Mild* COVID	0.390	0.227	0.070
10	HCQ with AZM	*severe* COVID	0.300	−0.119	0.065
100	HCQ	Control	0.505	0.230	0.085
100	HCQ	*Mild* COVID	0.450	0.159	0.090
100	HCQ	*severe* COVID	0.345	−0.075	0.080
100	HCQ with AZM	Control	0.630	0.317	0.075
100	HCQ with AZM	*Mild* COVID	0.555	0.220	0.075
100	HCQ with AZM	*severe* COVID	0.355	−0.05	0.070

Table 4.
Surrogate biomarker such as QT interval, T-peak and QRS duration of controlled, mild and severely infected COVID ventricle in response to various HCQ doses (1, 10 and 100 μM) alone or with 1 μM AZM [21].

similar ECG complexes (with positive widened T-waves) as that in usual pacing. The regular beat resumes after a long pause at 3.3 sec.

Further, on the inclusion of 1 μM AZM with each of the 1 μM, 10 μM and 100 μM HCQ config, the QT interval prolongs by 7.14%, 20% and 80% respectively, in the control ventricle as shown in **Figure 1**(iii). Likewise, the T-peak increases by 3.87%, 37.5% and 36.63% under AZM in combination with 1 μM, 10 μM and 100 μM HCQ respectively. However, the QRS duration remains the same in both 1μM and 10 μM HCQ, but increases by 7.14% in 100 μM HCQ. Additionally, PVCs arise due to the inclusion of PBs in the combination of 1 μM HCQ and AZM, and regular pulses resume at 1.6 sec. The occurrence of PVCs increases in the presence of PBs in 10 μM HCQ, as seen in **Figure 1**(iv). This effect is due to the change in repolarisation sequence of the cells, specifically occurring from endo to mid and epi. Regular pulses resume at 2.4 sec. Although no reentry is generated in the tissue, the appearance of PVCs is a precursor to the development of arrhythmia. This finding is in line with the Wang et al., [14], where a dosage of 10 μM HCQ prolonged the APD of cells but did not induce an arrhythmia in tissue on decreasing the pacing interval. Further, the combination of HCQ and AZM created arrhythmic activity. Although no arrhythmic event was generated in the presence of 100 μM HCQ, widened T-waves occurred. Such broad-based and symmetrical T-waves, usually with increased amplitude, are termed as hyperacute T-waves and often associated with a depressed ST are a sign of acute ischemia (**Figure 5**) [22].

In the mild COVID-19 scenario, the QT interval becomes shortened by 7.14% (0.325 sec), and the T-peak decreases by 34.48% while the QRS duration remains unchanged as shown in (**Figure 6(i)**). While using 1 μM HCQ, the model's outcome, Pseudo ECG's QT interval increases by 1.43% with a double notch T-peak of 0.124 mV and 0.110 mV. For the 10 μM, the pseudo-ECG prolongs the QT interval and increases the T-peak by 11.42% and 18.10%, respectively. When HCQ dosage is 100 μM, the QT interval raises by 35.71% with a 3.02% T-peak increase and 21.4% prolongation of QRS duration. However, in the case of 1 μM and 10 μM HCQ, QRS duration increases by 7.14%. In the arrhythmogenesis test, three reduced duration PBs are applied; when the first PB is applied; the mid and epi cells in the tissue start to repolarization due to the excitation from the previous beat, as a consequence, the wave propagates upward along with the endo and mid-layers, and lastly, it enters the epi layer of the cardiac tissue. Succeeding that, the wavefront repolarizes from the endo, mid and epi layer with the cells located at the top of the epi layer repolarizing last, resulting in an inverted T-wave. During the second PB excitation (0.8 sec), the wavefront depolarizes the endo and mid-layer but is not able to excite the epi layer cells as they are in a refractory state and this results in an ST-segment elevation in the ECG, as indicated in (**Figure 6**(ii)). For the last PB, yet another PVC occurs and then regular beats resume at 1.6 sec. In the case of 10 μM HCQ, due to the change in repolarization pattern, PVCs occur, yet they do not lead to the formation of re-entrant patterns. When PB's are applied in 100 μM HCQ setup, ECG complexes with widened T-waves are observed.

When AZM was supplemented with 1 μM HCQ, 10 μM HCQ and 100 μM HCQ, the QT interval prolongs by a percentage of 7.14, 18.57 and 65.71 respectively, under *mild* COVID conditions (**Figure 6**(iii)). Furthermore, the T-peak increases by about 31% in the combination of AZM and 10 μM HCQ or 100 μM HCQ in comparison to *mild* COVID while there is negligible effect in 1 μM HCQ. Even though the QRS duration remains unchanged for 1 μM and 10 μM, it increases by 7.14% in 100 μM

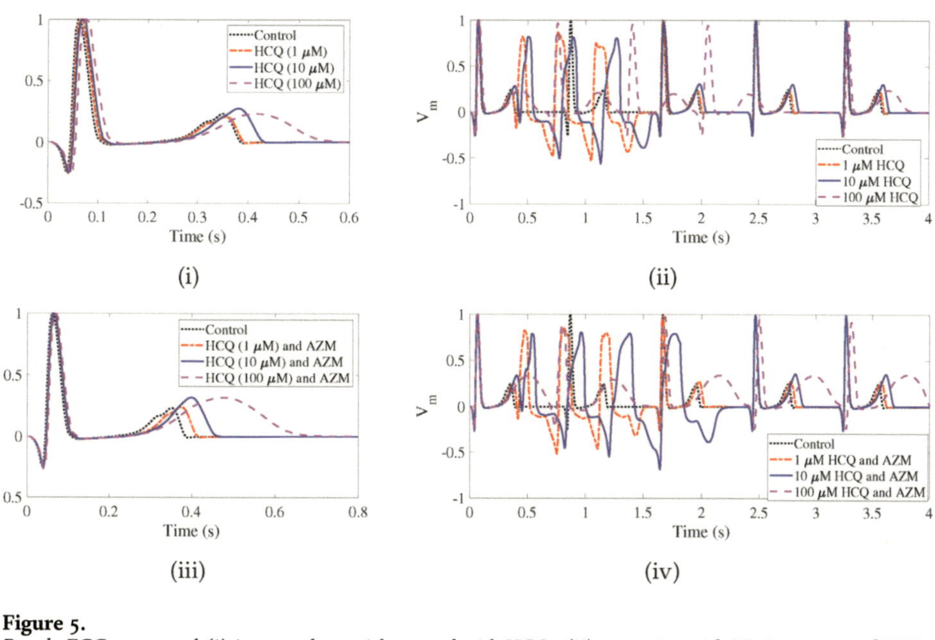

Figure 5.
Pseudo ECGs generated (i) in control ventricle treated with HCQ, (ii) on pacing with PBs in presence of HCQ, (iii) in control ventricle treated with HCQ and 1 μM of AZM, (iv) on pacing with PBs in presence of HCQ and 1 μM of AZM.

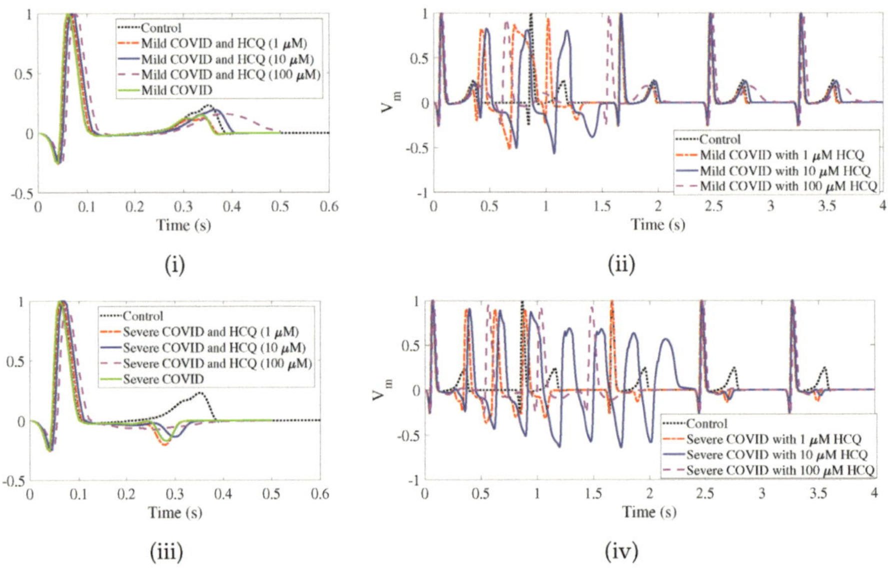

Figure 6.
Pseudo ECGs generated (i) in mild COVID-19 infected ventricle treated with HCQ, (ii) on pacing the mild COVID-19 infected ventricle with PBs with HCQ inhibition, (iii) in severe COVID-19 infected ventricle treated with HCQ, (iv) on pacing the severe COVID-19 infected ventricle tissue with PBs in presence of HCQ.

HCQ with 1 μM AZM. On pacing with PBs, PVCs occurred in both 1 μM HCQ and 10 μM HCQ conditions, and the regular pulses resume at 1.6 sec as shown in **Figure 6**(iv). When AZM is supplied with 100 μM HCQ and on applying PBs, no arrhythmic activity appeared in spite of the presence of the hyper-acute T-waves.

In *severe* COVID-19 configuration, the QT interval reduces by 21.48% (0.275 sec) with a negative T-wave peak of −0.17 mV and QT depression as shown in **Figure 6(v)**. This negative T-peak episode might be the representation of ischemia, which is in line with the clinical ECG recordings [23]. On treating with 1 μM HCQ, the QT interval reduces by 2.85% in comparison to severe COVID-19 and the negative T-peak increases by 15.51%. In contrast, under 10 μM HCQ, the QT interval increase by 4.28%, with a 14.22% reduction in T-peak. When the tissues are treated with 100 μM HCQ, the QT interval prolongs by 20%, with an immense reduction in the T-peak (i.e.) 40.98% in comparison to severe COVID-19. Here, the QRS duration is increased by 14.28% in 100 μM HCQ; while remaining unchanged at other dosages. In *severe* COVID-19, the inclusion of 1 μM HCQ and premature pacing sequence creates ECG complexes with increased negative T-peak amplitude due to the changes in the repolarisation pattern as seen in **Figure 2**(vi). The regular pulses are resumed after a long pause at 1.6 sec. In contrast, on including 10 μM HCQ and pacing the tissue with the first PB, the M-cells at the top of the tissue are still in the repolarising state. Therefore, the wave travels upwards along with the endo and mid-layer before entering the epi layer. This creates a change in the repolarisation pattern with endo cells repolarising first, followed by mid and epi cells. A similar activation pattern occurs on applying the second PB. When the third PB endures, the epi cells are repolarising; thus, the wavefront travels upwards along with the endo and mid-layer and re-enters the epi layer from the top. Further, the wavefront travels down along the epi layer and re-enters into the mid and endo layer. This reentrant activity creates upward and downward pointing QRS complexes, as shown in 6(vi) and the regular pacing resumes at 2.4 sec following the re-entry termination; for details, refer the voltage maps video1 provided in the Supplementary session. In the case of 100 μM HCQ, no arrhythmic activity or PVCs are observed, although flat T-waves occur,

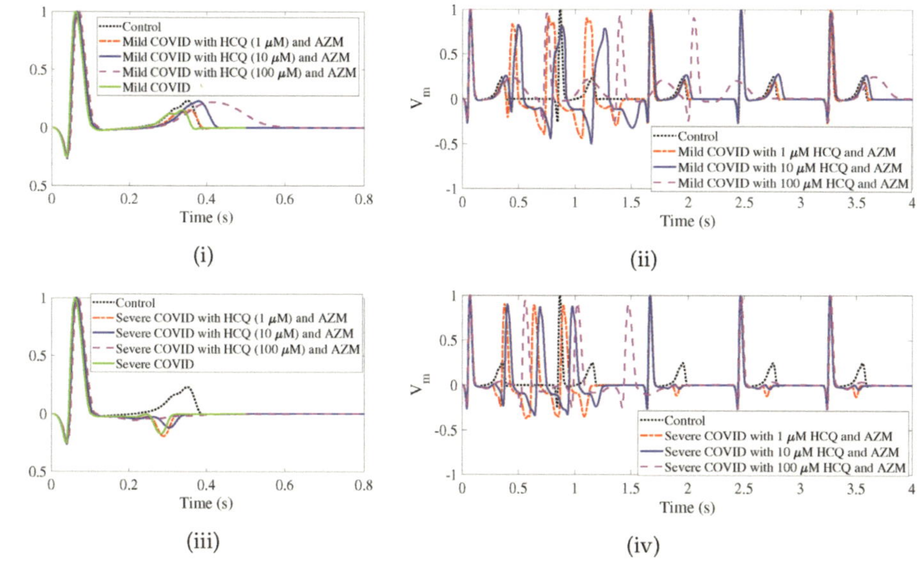

Figure 7.
Pseudo ECGs generated (i) in mild COVID-19 infected ventricle treated with HCQ and 1 μM AZM, (ii) on pacing the mild COVID-19 infected ventricle with PBs in presence of HCQ and 1 μM AZM, (iii)in severe COVID-19 infected ventricle treated with HCQ and 1 μM AZM, (iv) on pacing the severe COVID-19 infected ventricle tissue with PBs in presence of HCQ and 1 μM AZM.

representing the appearance of myocardial ischemia event [24] or hypokalemia [25]. The above result infers that an inverted T-wave morphology (representative of ischemia) can be a biomarker for *severe* COVID-19 screening.

On including AZM, as indicated in **Figure 6**(vii), the QT interval increases by 2.85%, 7.14% and 22.85% with 1 μM HCQ, 10 μM HCQ and 100 μM HCQ respectively in comparison to *severe* COVID. The T-peak increases by 10.34% in the combination of AZM and 1 μM HCQ while it decreases by 21.98% and 51.72% in 10 μM HCQ and 100 μM HCQ respectively. The QRS duration decreases by 7.14% remains in the combination of AZM and 1 μM or 10 μM HCQ whereas it is unchanged in combination with 100 μM HCQ. On pacing the tissue with PBS, PVCs are observed under 1 μM HCQ and 10 μM HCQ while under 100 μM HCQ, no significant change in the flattened T-waves is observed as seen in as seen in **Figure 6**(viii). The voltage maps video2 under 100 μM HCQ and AZM is provided in the Supplementary session (**Figure 7**).

5. Pacing sequence influence on arrhythmogenesis

In addition, to earlier pacing sequence, after the first beat is introduced, PBs are injected, under two condition, a) three unequal PBs with 800 msec (i.e., HR is 75 beats/min) pulse sequence, b) three equal PBs with 600 msec (i.e., HR is 100 beats/min), tachycardia pulse sequence. In each case, the first PBs duration is determined based on the refractory state and re-excitable property of bottom endo cells in the tissue. Further, the presence of PBs in mild and severe COVID-19 configurations for various HCQ dosages is applied to examine when an arrhythmia occurs.

Under mild COVID-19 and 1 μM HCQ conditions, three PBs are injected with reduced duration after the first regular beat. The mid and epi cells are still repolarizing when the first PB is applied; this causes the depolarization wave to travel upwards and the endo and mid-layers and later enter the epi layer. Following depolarization, repolarization occurs in the endo, mid and then epi layer, with the cells located at the top of the epi layer repolarizing lastly, leading to a premature ventricular complex (PVC). The depolarization wavefront from the second PB at 0.8-sec proceeds along with the endo and mid layer, however, it cannot excite the epi layer cells as they are in a refractory state, and this appears as an ST-segment elevation. Further, the third PB gives rise to another PVC and at 1.6 sec, the regular beats resume with notched T-waves. For 10 μM HCQ and mild cases, the three PBs give rise to PVCs due to the change in repolarization pattern, and wavefront reentry is absent. However, the QT interval and T-peak increase compared to control. ECG complexes with widened T-waves increased QT interval, and QRS duration is observed on pacing the tissue with three PBs under mild COVID-19 and 100 μM HCQ conditions. In severe COVID-19, the inclusion of 1 μM HCQ or 10 μM HCQ with three PBs for every 245 msec and 265 msec respectively give rise to PVCs with an increased negative/inverted T-peak. This result could be due to the repolarization pattern changes. However, in 100 μM HCQ conditions, no significant change is observed with similar ECG complexes occurring on applying three PBs at a pacing interval of 460 msec. The normal ECGs resumed at 1.2 sec in all three scenarios. Thus, the result inferred that an inverted T-wave morphology (representative of ischemia) could serve as a biomarker for severe COVID-19 conditions.

6. Limitation

In this study, we considered a 2D anisotropic transmural ventricular model, in which the entire mid-layer is composed of M-cells with longer APD. However, certain studies have disputed the presence of M-cells [26, 27] and others have debated that they form islands in the endo-mid interface [28, 29]. Here, arrhythmic patterns are generated through a premature pacing sequence. Like other few other studies, [16], here we had not considered using the cross-pacing sequence to simulate an arrhythmia, as the propagation pattern would then travel parallel along the entire length of the ventricle from endo, mid and epi, and it would not mimic the actual depolarisation pattern in the ventricle and thereby result in irregular pseudo-ECG wave. Another option is the generic Short-long-short (SLS) pacing sequences that can initiate TdP pattern [30], which is our future direction. In clinical ECG recordings, self-terminating re-entrant arrhythmia of few cycles may not be considered critical. However, the limited duration of the reentry generated here is due to the consideration of the 2D ventricle model. In a three-dimensional or whole heart model, sustainable ventricular arrhythmias may occur. Finally, we considered 1 μM, 10 μM, and 100 μM of HCQ and 1 μM AZM dosage due to the ionic current percentage variation reported by Wang et al., clinical study.

7. Conclusions

This study presents the first complete electrophysiological mechanism of COVID infected ventricle tissue with and without hypokalemia comorbidities and its responses to HCQ treatment. This model strategically allows more direct studies of ion channel perturbation from clinical observation of infected victims. This study's main conclusion is that when healthy cardiac tissue is infected by COVID, it engenders shorter QT interval, low amplitude or inverted T-waves and ST depression, which could be used as biomarkers. When treated with HCQ, in case of severe COVID-19, there is no significant adverse effect, but in mild COVID-19, QT interval prolongs and T-peak increases in ECG. Secondly, COVID-19 withal to the comorbid cardiac ventricle causes a slight QT interval elongation, notched T-waves in hypokalemia1, inverted T-waves in the presence of all severe hypoxia. In particular, the hypokalemic ventricle is prone to arrhythmia in the presence of COVID-19 and the addition of HCQ drug has no significant effects. Increasing the dosage of HCQ has the effect of prolonging the QT interval, and QRS duration and inclusion of AZM magnifies this effect. PVCs could be detected on pacing the tissue with PBs at lower doses of HCQ, and it led to the initiation of reentrant arrhythmia in *severe* COVID-19 conditions. Further, the pacing protocol also determines the appearance of reentry. Thus, the finding of this in-silico model could be considered for HCQ management in patients with pre-existing pathologies.

Conflict of interest

The authors declare no conflict of interest.

Nomenclature

I_{Na}	Sodium Current
I_{Kr}	Rapid delayed rectifier potassium Current
I_{Ks}	Slow delayed rectifier potassium Current
I_{K1}	Inward rectifier potassium Current
I_{CaL}	L-type Calcium Current

Abbreviations

HCQ	Hydroxychloroquine
ACE2	Angiotensin-Converting Enzyme 2
AZM	Azithromycin
APD	Action Potential Duration
ATP	Adenosine Triphosphate
ECG	Electrocardiogram
PB	Premature Beat
Endo	Endocardial Layer
Mid/M	Midmyocardial Layer
Epi	Epicardial Layer
PVC	Premature Ventricular Complex
SARS-Cov2	Severe Acute Respiratory Syndrome Coronavirus
FDA	Food and Drugs Administration
WHO	World Health Organization
TdP	Torsades de Pointes

Author details

Srinivasan Jayaraman[1*†] and Ponnuraj Kirthi Priya[2†]

1 Life Science Unit, Bio Computational Group, TATA Consultancy Services Limited, Portland, OR, USA

2 Life Science Unit, Bio Computational Group, TATA Consultancy Services Limited, Bangalore, India

*Address all correspondence to: srinivasa.j@tcs.com

† These authors contributed equally.

References

[1] Chen CY, Wang FL, Lin CC. Chronic hydroxychloroquine use associated with QT prolongation and refractory ventricular arrhythmia. Clinical Toxicology. 2006;44(2):173–175.

[2] Nord JE, Shah PK, Rinaldi RZ, Weisman MH. Hydroxychloroquine cardiotoxicity in systemic lupus erythematosus: a report of 2 cases and review of the literature. In: Seminars in arthritis and rheumatism. vol. 33. Elsevier; 2004. p. 336–351.

[3] Yao X, Ye F, Zhang M, Cui C, Huang B, Niu P, et al. In vitro antiviral activity and projection of optimized dosing design of hydroxychloroquine for the treatment of severe acute respiratory syndrome coronavirus 2 (SARS-CoV-2). Clinical Infectious Diseases. 2020.

[4] Dan Zhou SMD, Tong Q. COVID-19: a recommendation to examine the effect of hydroxychloroquine in preventing infection and progression. Journal of Antimicrobial Chemotherapy. 11 May 2020.

[5] Capel RA, Herring N, Kalla M, Yavari A, Mirams GR, Douglas G, et al. Hydroxychloroquine reduces heart rate by modulating the hyperpolarization-activated current If: Novel electrophysiological insights and therapeutic potential. Heart rhythm. 2015;12(10):2186–2194.

[6] Rodriguez B. Multiscale modeling and simulation investigation of variability and abnormalities in repolarization: Application to drug cardiotoxicity. In: 2010 Computing in Cardiology. IEEE; 2010. p. 257–260.

[7] Gautret P, Lagier JC, Parola P, Meddeb L, Mailhe M, Doudier B, et al. Hydroxychloroquine and azithromycin as a treatment of COVID-19: results of an open-label non-randomized clinical trial. International journal of antimicrobial agents. 2020:105949.

[8] Amrita X Sarkar DJC, Sobie EA. Exploiting mathematical models to illuminate electrophysiological variability between individuals. The Journal of Physiology;590.

[9] Mercuro NJ, Yen CF, Shim DJ, Maher TR, McCoy CM, Zimetbaum PJ, et al. Risk of QT Interval Prolongation Associated With Use of Hydroxychloroquine With or Without Concomitant Azithromycin Among Hospitalized Patients Testing Positive for Coronavirus Disease 2019 (COVID-19). JAMA cardiology. 2020.

[10] Li X, Hu C, Su F, Dai J, et al. Hypokalemia and clinical implications in patients with coronavirus disease 2019 (COVID-19). MedRxiv. 2020.

[11] He J, Wu B, Chen Y, Tang J, Liu Q, Zhou S, et al. Characteristic ECG manifestations in patients with COVID-19. Canadian Journal of Cardiology. 2020.

[12] Gattinoni L, Coppola S, Cressoni M, Busana M, Rossi S, Chiumello D. Covid-19 does not lead to a "typical" acute respiratory distress syndrome. American journal of respiratory and critical care medicine. 2020;(ja).

[13] Bennett CE, Anavekar NS, Gulati R, Singh M, Kane GC, Sandoval Y, et al. ST-segment Elevation, Myocardial Injury, and Suspected or Confirmed COVID-19 Patients: Diagnostic and Treatment Uncertainties. In: Mayo Clinic Proceedings. Elsevier; 2020. .

[14] Wang D, Hu B, Hu C, Zhu F, Liu X, Zhang J, et al. Clinical characteristics of 138 hospitalized patients with 2019 novel coronavirus–infected pneumonia in Wuhan, China. Jama. 2020;323(11): 1061–1069.

[15] White NJ, Watson JA, Hoglund RM, Chan XHS, Cheah PY, Tarning J. COVID-19 prevention and treatment: a critical analysis of chloroquine and hydroxychloroquine clinical pharmacology. PLoS medicine. 2020;17 (9):e1003252.

[16] Ten Tusscher KH, Panfilov AV. Alternans and spiral breakup in a human ventricular tissue model. American Journal of Physiology-Heart and Circulatory Physiology. 2006;291 (3):H1088–H1100.

[17] Priya PK, Reddy MR. Study of factors affecting the progression and termination of drug induced torsade de pointes in two dimensional cardiac tissue. Journal of electrocardiology. 2017;50(3):332–341.

[18] Shaw RM, Rudy Y. Electrophysiologic effects of acute myocardial ischemia: a theoretical study of altered cell excitability and action potential duration. Cardiovascular research. 1997;35(2):256–272.

[19] Clayton RH. Re-entry in a model of ischaemic ventricular tissue. In: 2010 Computing in Cardiology. IEEE; 2010. p. 181–184.

[20] Waldo A. Prevalence and Prognostic Significance of Short QT Interval in a Middle-Aged Finnish Population Anttonen O, Junttila MJ, Rissanen H, et al (P¨aij¨at-H¨ame Central Hosp, Lahti, Finland; Natl Public Health Inst, Helsinki; Univ of Helsinki; et al) Circulation 116: 714-720, 2007. Year Book of Cardiology. 2008; 2008:512–513.

[21] Wang G, Tian X, Lu CJ, Flores H, Maj P, Zhang K, et al. Mechanistic insights into ventricular arrhythmogenesis of hydroxychloroquine and azithromycin for the treatment of COVID-19. bioRxiv. 2020.

[22] Levis JT. ECG diagnosis: isolated posterior wall myocardial infarction. The Permanente Journal. 2015;19(4): e143.

[23] Hanna EB, Glancy DL. ST-segment depression and T-wave inversion: classification, differential diagnosis, and caveats. Cleveland Clinic journal of medicine. 2011;78(6):404.

[24] Morris F, Brady WJ. ABC of clinical electrocardiography: acute myocardial infarction—Part I. Bmj. 2002;324(7341): 831–834.

[25] Chua CE, Choi E, Khoo EY. ECG changes of severe hypokalemia. QJM: An International Journal of Medicine. 2018;111(8):581–582.

[26] Bryant SM, Wan X, Shipsey SJ, Hart G. Regional differences in the delayed rectifier current (I Kr and I Ks) contribute to the differences in action potential duration in basal left ventricular myocytes in guinea-pig. Cardiovascular research. 1998;40(2): 322–331.

[27] Rodriguez-Sinovas A, Cinca J, Tapias A, Armadans L, Tresanchez M, Soler-Soler J. Lack of evidence of M-cells in porcine left ventricular myocardium. Cardiovascular research. 1997;33(2):307–313.

[28] Antzelevitch C. M cells in the human heart. Circulation research. 2010;106(5):815–817.

[29] Glukhov AV, Fedorov VV, Lou Q, Ravikumar VK, Kalish PW, Schuessler RB, et al. Transmural Dispersion of Repolarization in Failing and Non Failing Human Ventricle. Circulation research. 2010;106(5):981.

[30] Sweeney MO, Ruetz LL, Belk P, Mullen TJ, Johnson JW, Sheldon T. Bradycardia pacing-induced short-long-short sequences at the onset of ventricular tachyarrhythmias: a possible mechanism of proarrhythmia? Journal of the American College of Cardiology. 2007;50(7):614–622.

Chapter 4

The Evolving Concept of Cardiac Conduction System Pacing

Iurii Karpenko, Dmytro Skoryi and Dmytro Volkov

Abstract

Cardiac pacing is an established treatment option for patients with bradycardia and heart failure. In the recent decade, there is an increasing scientific and clinical interest in the topic of direct His bundle pacing (HBP) and left bundle branch pacing (LBBP) as options for cardiac conduction system pacing (CSP). The concept of CSP started evolving from the late 1970s, passing several historical landmarks. HBP and LBBP used in CSP proved to be successful in small cohorts of patients with various clinical conditions, including binodal disease, atrioventricular blocks, and in patients with bundle branch blocks with indications for cardiac resynchronization therapy. The scope of this chapter is synthesis and analysis of works devoted to this subject, as well as representation of the author's experience in this topic. The chapter includes historical background, technical, anatomical, and clinical considerations of CSP, covers evidence base, discusses patient outcomes in line with the pros and cons of the abovementioned methods. The separate part describes practical aspects of different pacing modalities, including stages of the operation and pacemaker programming. The textual content of the chapter is accompanied by illustrations, ECGs, and intracardiac electrograms.

Keywords: His bundle pacing, left bundle branch pacing, cardiac pacing, conduction system pacing, interventricular septum, electrophysiology, cardiac resynchronization therapy

1. Introduction

Cardiac pacing from the right ventricular apical (RVA) site results in non-physiological ventricular activation, which leads to ventricular function impairment in a long-term perspective. Alternative pacing sites include right ventricular septal pacing (RVSP) and right ventricular (RV) outflow tract pacing; they are thought to be more beneficial to patients because of possibly better activation patterns than the RVA pacing. However, studies on pacing sites that are alternative to RVA are still contradictory as activation still relies on myocardial cell-to-cell conduction, thus does not prevent the development of pacing-induced cardiomyopathy [1]. Biventricular pacing (BVP) is a more favorable option than RVA pacing but still produces non-physiological activation patterns. The ideal physiological cardiac pacing requires sustained proximity to the intrinsic cardiac conduction system that preserves normal QRS complexes or even narrows QRS pattern in the bundle branch block (BBB) presence.

Direct conduction system pacing (CSP) becomes a frontier in the field of cardiac pacing, collecting evidence both from follow-up data and clinical case reports resulting in favor of His bundle (HB) pacing (HBP) and left bundle branch pacing (LBBP) as targets for His-Purkinje CSP. Although, it is necessary to mention that randomized clinical trials or meta-analyses that compare conventional pacing techniques to CSP are currently absent.

2. Historical landmarks

2.1 Predispositions for development

Permanent right ventricular pacing was firstly performed in humans on October 8th, 1958 by Swedish Surgeon Ake Senning. It was a breakthrough of that time, allowing to cope with Adams–Stokes syndrome to a 43-year-old man. Overall, this patient required 26 pacemakers to extend his life for 40 years and to live asymptomatically up to the age of 83 [2].

After 10 years from that date, in 1969, Narula, Sherlag proposed HBP using the electrophysiological catheter for HB stimulation. Authors also supposed a possibility of HB longitudinal dissociation.

More than 30 years passed since that time before Deshmukh et al. firstly implied this method in a group of patients of 12 with atrial fibrillation and indications for permanent cardiac pacing, "narrow" QRS complex, decreased left ventricular ejection fraction (LVEF) of 40% or less and NYHA III-IV [3]. For these purposes, the authors used standard electrodes with active fixation and modified stylet.

HBP was technically possible only in 66% of cases. The authors admitted a statistically significant increase in LVEF from 20 ± 9% to 31 ± 11% ($p < 0.01$). They supposed that the development of dedicated delivery systems for His-electrodes may turn an idea of more physiological cardiac pacing into reality, thus improving conventional RV pacing. However, this article reached the public at the time of BVP prosperity. BVP was proposed as a solution to tackle interventricular asynchronicity that progressively developed in scientific and practical aspects while being supported by the manufactures of cardiac pacemakers.

Numerous randomized clinical trials of cardiac resynchronization therapy (CRT) with the use of biventricular pacemakers and left ventricular epicardial pacing left HBP behind for more than 10 years. It was the first historical curiosity in HBP development.

2.2 Modern stage

At the same time, there was a rise in articles that analyzed predominantly retrospective data regarding HBP [4, 5]. The number of publications devoted to the HBP increases significantly since 2015. Among them are publications that analyze HBP in patients with atrioventricular (AV) block and sick sinus syndrome (SSS) [6]. Separate studies were dedicated to the comparison of HBP and RV pacing [7, 8], as well as to the evaluation of short-term and long-term outcomes of HBP [9].

A significant contribution to the topic was added by Vijayaraman et al. [6, 10] from Geisinger Heart Institute, USA, who demonstrated a technical possibility of HBP with the use of the 4.1 Fr Select Secure 3830 (Medtronic, USA) leads, which boosted the technical efficiency of HBP and expanded indications for it. It was the second curiosity in the HBP history because the abovementioned stylet-less pacing lead was initially developed about 20 years ago for permanent pacing in children with AV blocks, but not for the dedicated HBP.

3. His bundle pacing reasoning

3.1 Lead placement sites

Current approaches to the CSP base on the placement of the permanent pacing leads in the sites of the cardiac conduction system other than the RVA. CSP intends to overcome an asynchronous activation during pacing by producing the most physiologic activation pattern close to the one seen in the intrinsic conduction system. For that purpose, CSP leads may be implanted either at the HB or at the region of the left bundle branch (LBB) for different resynchronization strategies (**Figure 1**). The advantages and limitations of different strategies will be discussed later in the chapter.

3.2 Activation pattern

HBP has potential advantages in comparison to the CRT with the use of coronary sinus (CS) for left ventricular (LV) pacing [11]. LV pacing through CS cannot provide ideal resynchronization because of asynchronicity from the LV epicardial pre-excitation (**Figure 2**) [12]. Predominantly pacing comes from a lateral wall of the LV. The higher degree of asynchronicity can be seen through LV apical pacing and pacing in the areas with myocardial fibrotic scarring.

Both RV pacing and BVP change QRS pattern to a greater or lesser extent. Complete identically of QRS pattern to an intrinsic one differentiates HBP from the rest of pacing techniques [11]. Moreover, it is possible to completely or partly renew the intrinsic ventricular conduction in patients with BBBs by obtaining the normal width and form of the QRS complex [13, 14].

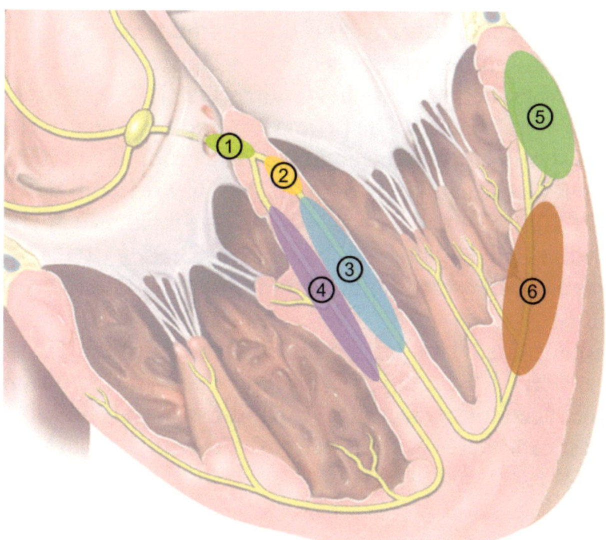

Figure 1.
Locations of the permanent lead placement for ventricular pacing along with strategies for cardiac resynchronization therapy. 1 – His bundle pacing; 2 – Left bundle branch pacing; 3 – Left septal pacing; 4 – Right septal pacing; 5 – Epicardial left ventricular pacing; 6 – Endocardial left ventricular pacing. Cardiac resynchronization therapy strategies: 1 – SINGLE SPOT (1, 2, 3, 4); 2 – CRT (4 + 5); 3 – HOT-CRT (1 + 5); 4. LOT-CRT (2, 3 + 5); 5. CSP-RV (2, 3 + 4). SINGLE SPOT = pacing from a single site, CRT = cardiac resynchronization therapy, HOT-CRT = His-optimized cardiac resynchronization therapy, LOT-CRT = left bundle branch-optimized cardiac resynchronization therapy, CSP-RV = conduction system pacing + right ventricular pacing.

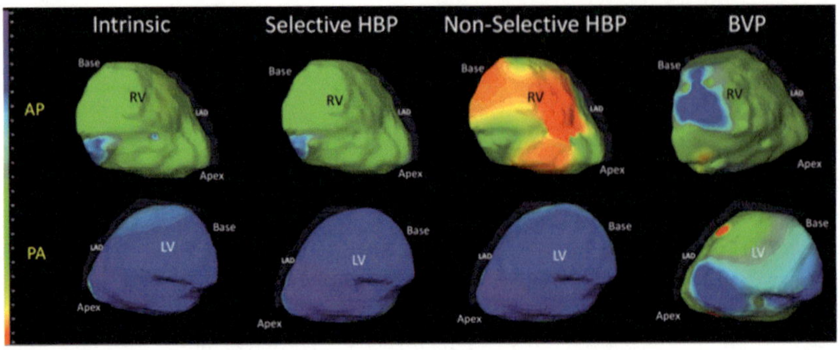

Figure 2.
Comparison of epicardial activation maps for intrinsic QRS, selective HBP, non-selective HBP, and BVP in a patient with normal QRS morphology and duration. The color scale on the left indicates the activation times. Activation from the selective HBP is identical to intrinsic activation. Activation from the non-selective HBP is identical to the intrinsic activation for LV, but evidence of pre-excitation can be seen for RV in the basal and mid areas, which indicates the capture RV myocardium alongside the HB. The activation pattern in the case of BVP is different from an intrinsic one. Differences between selective and non-selective HBP will be discussed later in the chapter. AP – Anterior–posterior projection, PA – Posterior–anterior projection, LAD – Left anterior descending artery.

3.3 Clinical implications

Clinical interest in the HBP significantly increased in the previous 5 years.

The largest study regarding the clinical of HBP compared to the RV pacing was published in 2018 [7]. Patients requiring pacemaker implantation were included in the study between 2013 and 2016. HBP was performed in consecutive patients at 1 hospital, while other patients received RV pacing at a sister hospital. A total of 765 people underwent pacemaker implantation: RV pacing in 433 patients and HBP in 332 patients. HBP was technically successful in 304 patients (92%). The mean follow-up duration for the entire cohort was 725 + 423 days.

Implant characteristics, heart failure hospitalization (HFH), upgrades to BVP and all-case mortality were tracked. The primary endpoint of death, HFH, or upgrade to BiVP was significantly reduced in the HBP group (83 of 332 patients [25%]) compared to RVP (137 of 433 patients [32%]; hazard ratio [HR]: 0.71; 95% confidence interval [CI]: 0.534 to 0.944; $p = 0.02$). The incidence of HFH was significantly reduced in HBP (12.4% vs. 17.6%; HR: 0.63; 95% CI: 0.430 to 0.931; $p = 0.02$). There was a trend toward reduced mortality in HBP (17.2% vs. 21.4%, respectively; $p = 0.06$).

From the abovementioned data, it is possible to conclude that HBP can be an alternative to conventional RV pacing in clinical practice while improving patient outcomes, taking into account the technical capabilities of the clinic and accumulated experience. Best candidates for HBP are patients with AV blocks, "narrow" QRS, and impaired LV function [15–17].

4. His bundle pacing in different patient groups

4.1 Patients with indications for CRT

HBP is more frequently used nowadays as an alternative to conventional RV pacing in patients with intraventricular conduction disturbances and indications for CRT. The idea of overcoming distal His-Purkinje system injury with the help of HBP and thus renew normal ventricular conduction seems very appealing [10].

Several groups of patients with intraventricular blocks that were previously treated as distal His-Purkinje injury can successfully restore conduction despite BBB [4, 13, 18–21].

An exact mechanism of QRS complex normalization in these cases is not fully understood. A hypothesis of functional longitudinal dissociation in HB that is the most widespread nowadays for explaining HBP efficiency in BBB was initially proposed by Kaufman R. and Rothberger C in the already distant 1919 [22]. The core of the hypothesis is that there are fibers inside the HB that conduct pacing impulses to the left and right bundle branches, being predominantly isolated from each other. Because of that, damage of these fibers in one of the HBs results in HB branch blocks [23]. It means that His-Purkinje system fibers may be blocked proximally, not distally inside the interventricular septum (IVS), and this block can be corrected with direct HBP.

Basing on the HB anatomy, the current amplitude for pacing specialized HB branch fibers (partially isolated by connective tissue) may be relatively high and involve neighboring myocardial areas [24, 25]. It is necessary to discuss the mechanisms of the non-selective HBP [26, 27]. In non-selective HBP, besides the activation of the HB fibers with block overcoming, additional areas of the adjacent myocardium (mostly septal part of the RV, rarely basal parts of the LV) may be activated.

The main aim of the research conducted by Huang W. et al. was to assess the efficacy of HBP to correct LBB block (LBBB) and long-term clinical outcomes with HBP in patients with heart failure (HF) [13]. Permanent HBP leads were implanted in HB under the guidance of ECG criteria for LBBB correction and pacing threshold <3.5 V / 0.5 ms or 3.0 V / 1 ms. Left ventricular ejection fraction (LVEF), left ventricular end-systolic volume (LVESV), pacing parameters, and NYHA class was assessed during a follow-up. HBP was performed in 74 patients (mean age 69.6 ± 9.2 years and 43 men). LBBB correction was reached in 72 patients (97.3%). 56 patients (75.7%) had adequate pacing thresholds during HB lead implantation. Lead implantation wasn't performed in 18 patients because of a lack of LBBB correction (n = 2) or high pacing threshold for LBBB correction (n = 16). An average follow-up was 37 (range 15.0–48.7) months. Follow-up exceeded 3 years in 30 patients with HBP. Patients had an increase in LVEF from baseline32.4 ± 8.9% to 55.9 ± 10.7% ($p < 0.001$), LVESV decreased from a baseline of 137.9 ± 64.1 mL to 52.4 ± 32.6 mL ($p < 0.001$) and NYHA Class improvement from baseline 2.73 ± 0.58 to 1.03 ± 0.18 ($p < 0.001$). The pacing threshold required for LBBB correction remained the same: 2.13 ± 1.19 V / 0.5 ms during a procedure and 2.29 ± 0.92 V / 0.5 ms at a 3-year follow-up ($p > 0.05$). The conclusions are as follows: HBP with LBBB resolution can be seen in 76% of patients and accompanied by a significant improvement of LV contraction properties. On the other hand, almost a quarter of patients cannot overcome LBBB while performing HBP; the question remains opened which technique should be considered next after HBP failure.

Close results were obtained by Ajijola O. et al. [28]. Selective HBP was successful in 16 patients (76%) out of 21 patients with LBBB. It lead to a significant decrease in the QRS complex duration from 180 ± 23 ms to 129 ± 13 ms ($p < .0001$) and LVEF improvement from 27% ± 10–41% ± 13% ($p < .001$) during a 12-month follow-up.

Sharma et al. performed HBP in candidates for CRT, to whom it was technically impossible to achieve LV epicardial pacing, or to the ones who were non-responders to a conventional CRT. HBP was technically successful in 95 patients out of 106 (90%). The mean follow-up period was 14 months. It was marked a significant decrease of QRS duration from 157 ± 33 ms to 117 ± 18 ms ($p = .0001$), an increase in LVEF from 30 ± 10% to 43 ± 13% ($p = .0001$), and NYHA Class improvement from 2.8 ± 0.5 to 1.8 ± 0.6 ($p = .0001$).

HBP nowadays is considered as an alternative to a conventional BVP in patients with LBBB and broad QRS complexes in addition to chronic ventricular pacing with heart failure and ventricular asynchrony [18, 19, 29–32].

However, HBP not always leads to a significant decrease of a ventricular complex. An aim to improve HBP results with the help of additional lead implantation through the coronary sinus to pace LV was set in His-optimized CRT (HOT-CRT) trial to reach a maximum possible resynchronization. This trial demonstrated a possibility of HBP optimization via this additional lead to LV through coronary sinus [33].

HOT-CRT was applied in 27 patients (mean age 72 ± 15 years): 17 with LBBB, 5 with intraventricular blocks, 5 with chronic RV pacing. HOT-CRT protocol was successfully run in 25 patients out of 27. The initial QRS width of 183 ± 27 ms was significantly reduced to 162 ± 17 ms for BVP and 151 ± 24 ms for HBP ($p < .0001$). With HOT-CRT protocol (His pacing lead implantation + LV pacing through coronary sinus), QRS length decreased even more to 120 ± 16 ms ($p < .0001$). Mean follow-up was 14 ± 10 months. LVEF increased from 24 ± 7% to 38 ± 10% ($p < .0001$), and NYHA Class was improved from 3.3 to 2.04. Clinical responders were 21 out of 25 patients (84%), and echocardiographic responders were 23 out of 25 patients (92%).

HOT-CRT trial demonstrated a possibility of electrical resynchronization improvement in patients with indications for CRT and suboptimal HBP by adding LV stimulation site through the coronary sinus.

The most common location for LBBB – is a left part of the HB. HBP eliminates LBBB on this level in 94% of cases. In the case of a more distal location of LBBB, correction is possible in 62% of cases. When the His-Purkinje system is intact on the level of IVS, LBBB correction with HBP does not take place.

In the clinical practice, preferable locations of the LBBB for HBP are left-sided proximal HB fibers blocks with a possibility of activation of the latent distal His-Purkinje system.

4.2 Patients with RBBB

Positive hemodynamical and clinical effects of BVP are limited in patients with right bundle branch block (RBBB). Permanent HBP is proposed as an option for resynchronization therapy in 39 patients with RBBB and low LVEF who had indications for CRT [21]. HBP was an initial strategy for them or a "rescue" strategy in a case of unsuccessful implantation of the epicardial lead for LV pacing.

Selective HBP was successful in 37 patients out of 39 (95%); however, a markable reduction in QRS duration was reached in 78% of cases. HB pacing thresholds for RBBB correction were 1.4 ± 0.7 V / 1 ms. Mean follow-up was 15 ± 23 months. A significant reduction in QRS length from 158 ± 24 ms to 127 ± 17 ms was achieved. LVEF improved from 31 ± 10% to 39 ± 13% ($p = .004$), and NYHA Class was decreased from 2.8 ± 0.6 to 2 ± 0.7 ($p = .0001$). The notable increase in pacing threshold was in 3 cases.

This research concluded that permanent HBS was associated with shortening QRS duration in patients with RBBB and decreased LVEF.

5. His bundle pacing limitations

5.1 Implantation site

The main boundary for the wide adoption of HBP is a relatively small area for pacing lead implantation into the cardiac conduction system with an appropriate pacing threshold. As a result, physicians experience lengthening of the procedure time and an increase in fluoroscopy exposure compared to conventional RV pacing. These problems tend to decrease with an accumulation of physician's experience. Nevertheless, even experienced physicians in high-volume centers perform HBP by 27% longer than RV pacing (70 mins and 55 mins) while increasing fluoroscopy time by 39% (10.3 mins and 7.4 mins) [34, 35].

Further improvements in implantation tools will help overcome technical limitations, but even in this case, procedure and fluoroscopy time will remain lengthier than for RV pacing [7].

5.2 Pacing thresholds

Another disadvantage of HBP – higher pacing thresholds and lesser energy efficiency that leads to the earlier cardiac pacemaker battery discharge. An increase in pacing threshold was observed in post-operational period for HBP compared to RV pacing: 1.30 V + 0.85 V for HBP and 0.59 V + 0.42 V for RV pacing. It resulted in a necessity for early pacemaker replacement in 3 out of 75 patients from the HBP group [7].

5.3 Lead fixation

Lead instability is another problem for HBP, which increases the probability of lead dislocation in the post-operational period despite the active lead fixation type [4, 8, 23, 27]. According to the data from Geisinger Institute, 4.2% of patients required lead correction after performing HBP [7].

5.4 Summary

Summing up data of HBP in patients with indications for CRT, it becomes possible to conclude that HBP leads to adequate cardiac resynchronization in 70–92% of cases, resulting in shortening of QRS complex compared to BVP and decreasing required time for the procedure.

Even though the solid theoretical background and practical applicability among experienced physicians, HBP cannot fully replace conventional BVP nowadays. HBP limitations include higher pacing thresholds, lower R-wave amplitude, and probable difficulties with ventricular signal sensing. On the other hand, there is also a possibility of hypersensitivity to far-field P-waves signals. Lead instability in continuous pacing is another point of concern, along with long-term effects of HBP because of potentially damaging influence on the distal structures of the His–Purkinje system.

Data from upcoming randomized clinical trials may remove the ambiguity in HBP [30, 32]. There is also a need for direct comparison of HBP to RV pacing and conventional multifocal BVP. Additional research may answer further questions regarding HBP complications and mechanisms of non-selective HBP. Could non-selective HBP be treated as an alternative to selective HBP? And what problems may arise during lead extraction?

Much work remains to be done with conducting thoroughly planned randomized clinical trials that will evaluate the potential of HBP in cardiac pacing.

6. Anatomical considerations for His bundle pacing

Knowledge of anatomical and physiological properties of cardiac conduction system, and HB in particular, is required for performing successful lead implantation for further HBP. Significant contribution to this topic was added by Kawashima T., Sasaki H. in 2005, who described relationship of the HB to the membranous part of the IVS based on the autopsy material of 105 subjects [25]. Authors outlined three anatomical variations of HB.

6.1 Normal atrioventricular bundle

The normal variant (type I) was in 49 subjects out of 105 (46.7%). The atrioventricular bundle (the HB) coursed along the lower border of the membranous part of the IVS and was covered by a thin layer of common myocardial fibers spanning from the muscular part to the membranous part of the IVS (**Figure 3**). Fusion phenomenon was seen during HBP in this anatomical variation, or non-selective HBP in higher current amplitude and selective HBP in lower current amplitude during pacing.

6.2 Deep-seated atrioventricular bundle

Deep-seated HB (type II) was found in 34 subjects out of 105 (32.4%). The atrioventricular bundle is clearly distinguished from the membranous part of the IVS and lays within the muscular portion of the IVS (**Figure 4**). In such cases, even in the clear identification of HB signal, it is a rare occurrence of adequate HBP.

6.3 Naked atrioventricular bundle

Naked HB (type III) was found in 22 subjects out of 105 (21%). It is located predominantly beneath the endocardium, and there is no overlay of muscle fibers (**Figure 5**). Possibly, it is the best type for HBP.

6.4 Summary

Thus, HB can be accessible for HBP in at least 68% of cases based on the data from the abovementioned study. Unfortunately, no technology nowadays can define the anatomical variant of HB before the lead implantation.

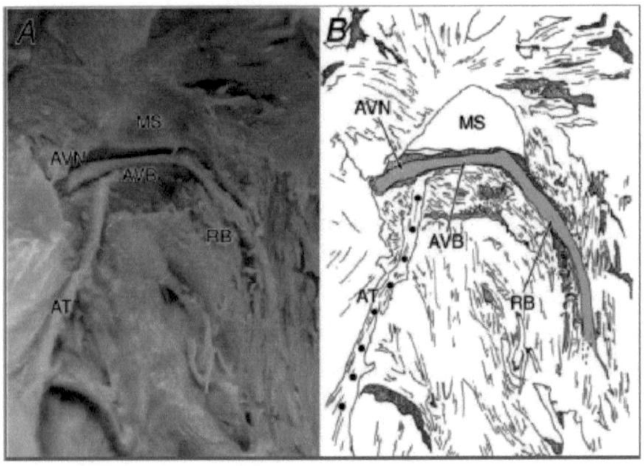

Figure 3.
HB of type I. A – Anatomical substrate; B – Graphical representation; AT - attachment of tricuspid valve; AVB - atrioventricular bundle; AVN - atrioventricular node; RB - right branch; MS - membranous part of the interventricular septum (Kawashima and Sasaki [25]).

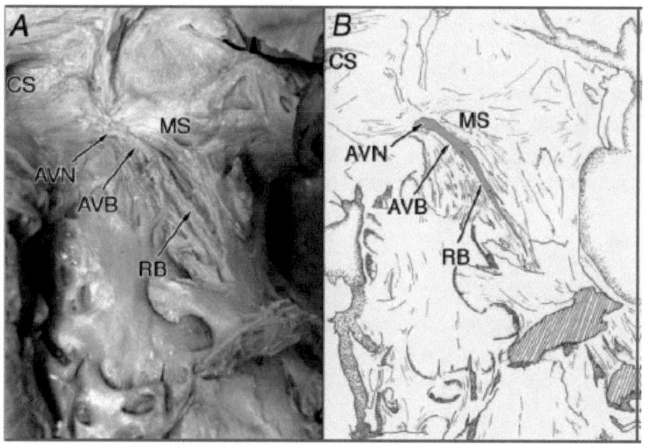

Figure 4.
HB of type II. A – Anatomical substrate; B – Graphical representation; AT - attachment of tricuspid valve; AVB - atrioventricular bundle; AVN - atrioventricular node; RB - right branch; MS - membranous part of the interventricular septum; CS - coronary sinus (Kawashima and Sasaki [25]).

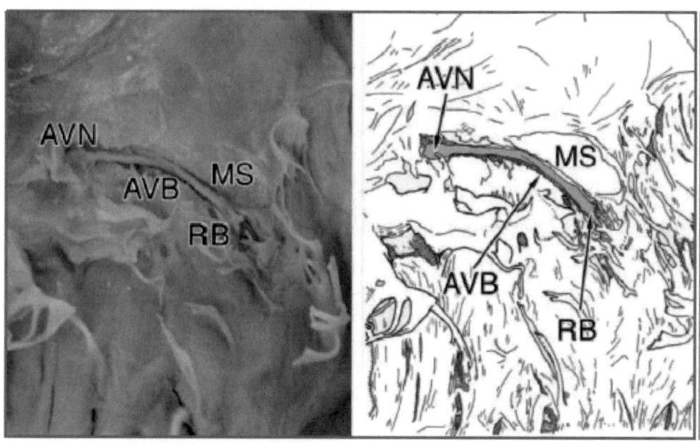

Figure 5.
HB of type III. AVB - atrioventricular bundle; AVN - atrioventricular node; RB - right branch; MS - membranous part of the interventricular septum (Kawashima and Sasaki [25]).

7. Practical recommendations for His bundle pacing

7.1 First stage. Venous access

For venous access, we preferably puncture left axillary vein. Usually, we enter with a short peel-away regular 7F sheath as it is congruent with advanced further C315 His catheter. While having a C315 catheter in RA, we try to place a guiding wire in RV. It advantages smooth guiding of C315 catheter to RV and avoids tip damaging during tricuspidal valve crossing. Afterward, the system withdrawing to the basal septal region is easier than penetrating forward.

7.2 Second stage. His bundle mapping

After the lead introducer system is positioned in a supposed projection of HB, signal mapping of HB starts from the distal tip of the lead to register unipolar or bipolar signal. For this purpose, a standard electrophysiological system can be used and/or PSA 3 signal analyzer and Medtronic programmer. It is advised to apply atrial channel for HB mapping as it is more sensitive. The cathode is

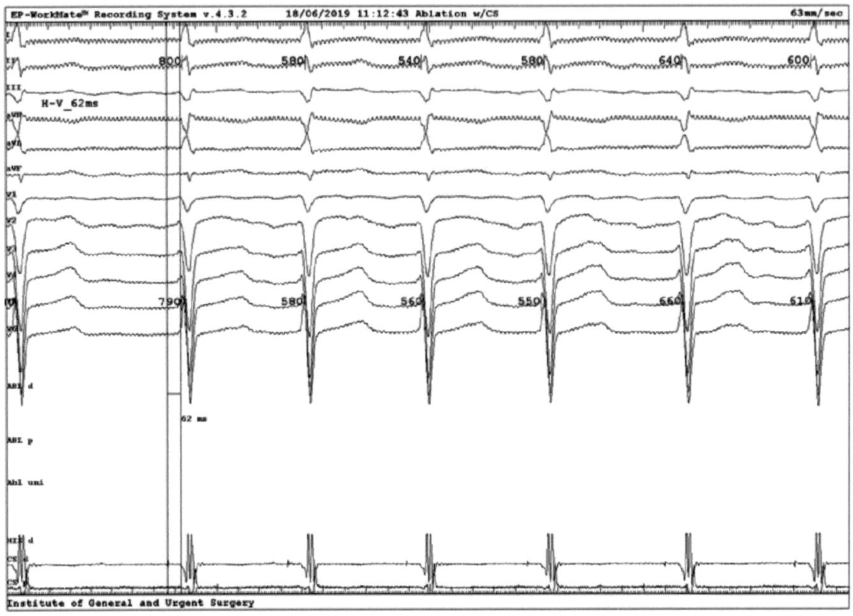

Figure 6.
HB mapping (total gain – 5000, filtration rate – 500 Hz).

connected to the distal tip and anode to the skin. After that, an accurate search of HB potentials starts. It is necessary to point out that the distal electrode (Helix) is in an active position what complicates the overall system manipulation; however, it is possible to map with Helix placed slightly inside the lumen of the delivery system (**Figures 6** and 7).

After HB mapping, it is necessary to know the main maneuvers with C 315 His introducer. For fluoroscopic visualization, RAO 15–30 position is used. Clockwise

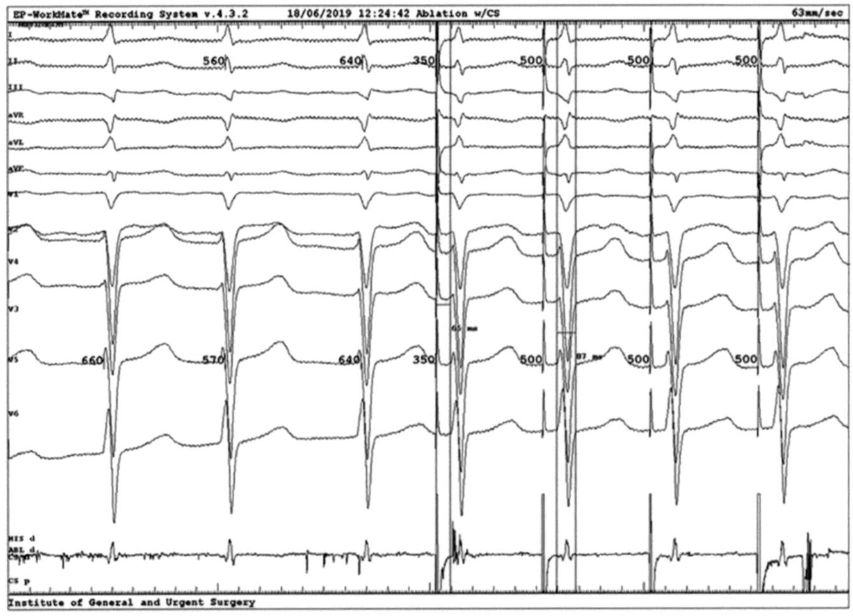

Figure 7.
HB mapping.

introducer rotation with an electrode inside turns its tip forward and upwards relative to the IVS. Counterclockwise introducer rotation directs it backwards, closer to the tricuspid valve.

C 315 His introducer is advanced maximally further through an electrode after identification of the HB signal. It adds additional stability to the system before lead implantation (screwing). His lead implantation is performed after HB signal assessment relative to the atrial and ventricular signals (**Figure 7**).

In a case when it is not possible to register discrete HB potential, the pace-mapping technique may be applied beginning with high amplitudes (5–10 V / 1 ms) with identification of the pacing threshold for RV and HB. This technique is especially useful for conducting HBP in patients with AV blocks.

7.3 Third stage. Lead implantation

Lead implantation starts with both operator's hands for clockwise rotation: 4–5 rotations with slight pressure on lead in a forward direction. Meanwhile assistant supports a delivery system in a necessary position (usually performing anticlockwise movements for pushing introducer and lead perpendicular to the implantation site). Additional rotations may be needed based upon tactic feelings and fluoroscopy. After fixation, the lead is pointed frontward while the introducer is retracted 3–5 cm backward, creating a moderate 'insurance' loop and evaluating lead fixation stability.

In the experimental post-mortem study, M. Jastrzebski et al. distinguished 3 types of lead behavior during deep septal implantation – entanglement, drill-effect, and screwdriver effect [36]. These behaviors depend on endo-myocardial tissue characteristics, positioning angle relative to the cardiac wall, and the way of screwing. Recognition of these behaviors might help to achieve successful penetration without complications and unnecessarily prolong attempts.

7.4 Fourth stage. His bundle pacing testing

R-wave amplitude test is performed afterward. Because of the thin myocardial layer in this region, acceptable values for appropriate R-wave sensing are more than 1–2 mV, which usually provides enough safety margin from far-field atrial and His signals oversensing. This makes use of pacemakers with maximum ventricular sensing of 0.5 mV more reasonable.

QRS complex assessment in standard 12-lead ECG with relatively high amplitude and duration of the pacing impulse (5 V / 1 ms) is the next step. A threshold test is conducted with a gradual decrease of the pacing impulse amplitude. It is necessary to define the threshold of selective HBP and RV pacing. The acceptable HBP threshold is less than 2.5 V / 1 ms. HBP threshold may decrease within 10–20 mins after implantation due to a decrease in an acute HB fibers traumatic damage.

An important prognostic factor is a change between selective and non-selective HBP in response to different pacing outputs. If decreasing a pacing output lead to a transition from non-selective to selective HBP, it is a strong predictor of a favorable outcome because the active electrode part is within the conduction system. The opposite sequence points out a more remote position from HB, and further considerations should be taken into account.

7.5 Fifth stage. Introducer extraction

For introducer extraction, a standard set of knives is used. The presence of a "secure" loop is mandatory before the introducer extraction; it provides sustainability to the lead. Extraction is guided by fluoroscopy to control the lead position.

Unfortunately, delivery and extraction systems are not the perfect ones. Because of that, it is necessary to be prepared for accurate delivery system dissection with small scissors.

After introducer extraction, there is an additional check of the ventricular signal amplitude and pacing thresholds for bipolar/monopolar configuration. Monopolar sensing is inadvisable in pacemaker-dependent patients (risk of atrial oversensing).

7.6 Sixth stage. Atrial lead implantation and pacemaker placement

Implantation of the atrial lead is conventionally performed in the right atrial appendage or the interatrial septum (**Figure 8**). Atrial and ventricular sensing should be no less than 0.45 mV.

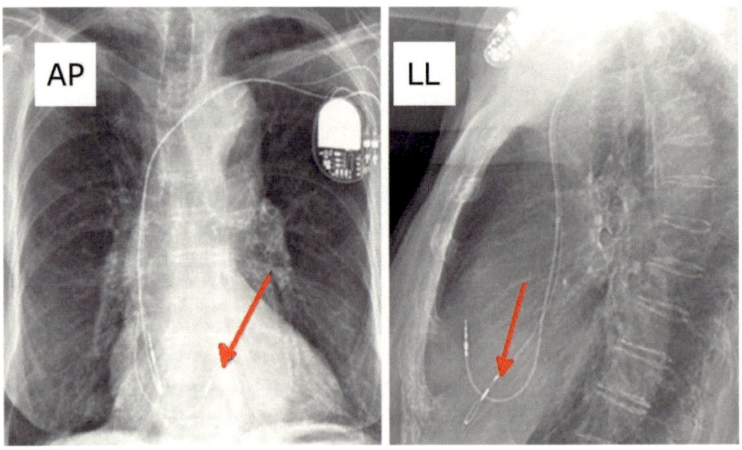

Figure 8.
Final lead and pacemaker positioning in HBP. Red arrow points at the HB pacing lead (AP LL view).

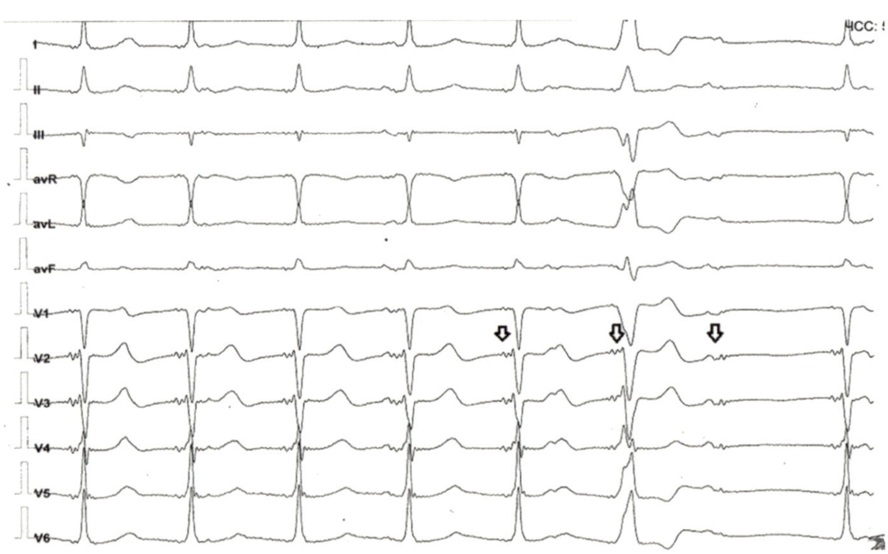

Figure 9.
Detection of the pacing threshold for HB. Asynchronous bipolar stimulation at 90 bpm. The first arrow marks the last QRS complex conducted through HB – Pacing threshold for HB. QRS width is 89 ms. the next QRS complex is a deformed one; its width is 167 ms – Pacing threshold for RV myocardium (second arrow). The third arrow points non-response spike.

In the presence of an initially high pacing threshold for HB, it is recommended to consider pacemakers with prolonged longevity.

7.7 Seventh stage. Programming

While programming a pacing amplitude, it is necessary to consider a probability of a significant rise in pacing threshold in a subacute period in 10% of cases. Non-selective HBP is a predominant pacing type among the patients and, because of probable lower pacing thresholds for myocardium versus HB, adequate pacing amplitude should be programmed 1.5–2 times higher than the HBP threshold (**Figure 9**). Myocardial capture is reserved as a back-up in case of HBP failure.

While programming an AV delay, the time of conducting potential through HB should be considered (H-V interval on electrogram). AV delay is shortened by the duration of this interval (~ 40–70 ms).

Additional attention should be paid to the hypersensitivity for the far-field atrial signal.

8. Conclusion

CSP nowadays becomes even more innovative. HBP and LBB pacing made continuous pacing even more physiologic in certain groups of patients with bradycardias and intraventricular conduction disturbances by restoring conduction close to the native one. A possibility to implant leads in the HB, and LBB creates new options for conducting CRT with such configurations as HOT-CRT or LOT-CRT for patients with corresponding indications. With improvements in HBP tools and accumulation of the individual experience, HBP will become one of the principal methods for bradycardia pacing in patients with intraventricular conduction disturbances and heart failure.

Conflict of interest

Nothing to declare.

Abbreviations

AP	anteroposterior
AV	atrioventricular
BBB	bundle branch block
BVP	biventricular pacing
CRT	cardiac resynchronization therapy
CS	coronary sinus
CSP	conduction system pacing
HB	His bundle
HBP	His bundle pacing
HF	heart failure
HFH	heart failure hospitalization
HOT-CRT	His-optimized CRT
IVS	intervetricular septum
LBB	left bundle branch
LBBB	left bundle branch block

LBBP	left bundle branch pacing
LL	left lateral
LOT-CRT	left bundle branch-optimized CRT
LV	left ventricle
LVEF	left ventricular ejection fraction
LVESV	left ventricular end-systolic volume
RAO	right anterior oblique
RBBB	right bundle branch block
RV	right ventricle
RVA	right ventricular apex
RVSP	right ventricular septal pacing
SSS	sick sinus syndrome

Author details

Iurii Karpenko[1], Dmytro Skoryi[2] and Dmytro Volkov[2]*

1 Department of Internal Medicine and Cardio-Vascular Pathology, Odessa National Medical University, Odessa, Ukraine

2 Department for Ultrasound and Instrumental Diagnostics with EP Lab, Zaycev V.T. Institute of General and Urgent Surgery of National Academy of Medical Science of Ukraine, Kharkiv, Ukraine

*Address all correspondence to: volkov@hearthealth.pro

References

[1] Ng AC, Allman C, Vidaic J, Tie H, Hopkins AP, Leung DY. Long-term impact of right ventricular septal versus apical pacing on left ventricular synchrony and function in patients with second- or third-degree heart block. Am J Cardiol. 2009;103(8):1096-1101. DOI: 10.1016/j.amjcard.2008.12.029

[2] Cooley DA. In memoriam. Tribute to Ake Senning, pioneering cardiovascular surgeon. Tex Heart Inst J. 2000;27(3):234-235.

[3] Deshmukh P, Casavant DA, Romanyshyn M, Anderson K. Permanent, direct His-bundle pacing: a novel approach to cardiac pacing in patients with normal His-Purkinje activation. Circulation. 2000;101(8): 869-877. DOI: 10.1161/01.cir.101.8.869

[4] Lustgarten DL, Calame S, Crespo EM, Calame J, Lobel R, Spector PS. Electrical resynchronization induced by direct His-bundle pacing. Heart Rhythm. 2010;7(1):15-21. DOI: 10.1016/j.hrthm.2009.09.066

[5] Occhetta E, Bortnik M, Marino P. Permanent parahisian pacing. Indian Pacing Electrophysiol J. 2007;7(2):110-125. Published 2007 Apr 1.

[6] Vijayaraman P, Dandamudi G. How to Perform Permanent His Bundle Pacing: Tips and Tricks. Pacing Clin Electrophysiol. 2016;39(12):1298-1304. DOI: 10.1111/pace.12904

[7] Abdelrahman M, Subzposh FA, Beer D, et al. Clinical Outcomes of His Bundle Pacing Compared to Right Ventricular Pacing. J Am Coll Cardiol. 2018;71(20):2319-2330. DOI: 10.1016/j.jacc.2018.02.048

[8] Sharma PS, Dandamudi G, Naperkowski A, et al. Permanent His-bundle pacing is feasible, safe, and superior to right ventricular pacing in routine clinical practice. Heart Rhythm. 2015;12(2):305-312. DOI: 10.1016/j.hrthm.2014.10.021

[9] Zanon F., Marcantoni L., Pastore G., Baracca E., Aggio S., Carraro M., Picariello C., Lanza D., Giatti S., Rinuncini M., Galasso M. P., D'elia K., Roncon L., Conte L. His bundle pacing in BBB patients: outcomes over a long-term follow-up. Europace. 2018. Vol. 20, N suppl_1. P. i2–i3.

[10] Vijayaraman P, Dandamudi G, Worsnick S, Ellenbogen KA. Acute His-Bundle Injury Current during Permanent His-Bundle Pacing Predicts Excellent Pacing Outcomes. Pacing Clin Electrophysiol. 2015;38(5):540-546. DOI: 10.1111/pace.12571

[11] Arnold AD, Shun-Shin MJ, Keene D, et al. His Resynchronization Versus Biventricular Pacing in Patients With Heart Failure and Left Bundle Branch Block. J Am Coll Cardiol. 2018;72(24):3112-3122. DOI: 10.1016/j.jacc.2018.09.073

[12] Arnold A, Shun-Shin M, Keene D, et al. Left ventricular activation time and pattern are preserved during both selective and non-selective His pacing (abstr). Heart Rhythm 2016;13:S342. DOI: 10.1016/j.hroo.2021.08.001

[13] Huang W, Su L, Wu S, et al. Long-term outcomes of His bundle pacing in patients with heart failure with left bundle branch block. Heart. 2019;105(2):137-143. DOI: 10.1136/heartjnl-2018-313415

[14] Lewis AJM, Foley P, Whinnett Z, Keene D, Chandrasekaran B. His Bundle Pacing: A New Strategy for Physiological Ventricular Activation [published correction appears in J Am Heart Assoc. 2019 Jun 4;8(11):e002310]. J Am Heart Assoc. 2019;8(6):e010972. DOI: 10.1161/JAHA.118.010972

[15] Curtis AB. Will His Bundle Pacing Make Cardiac Resynchronization Therapy Obsolete?. Circulation. 2018;137(15):1546-1548. DOI: 10.1161/CIRCULATIONAHA.117.031787

[16] Deshmukh P. His Bundle Pacing: Concept to Reality. Card Electrophysiol Clin. 2018;10(3):453-459. DOI: 10.1016/j.ccep.2018.05.007

[17] Upadhyay GA, Tung R. His Bundle Pacing for Cardiac Resynchronization. Card Electrophysiol Clin. 2018;10(3):511-517. DOI: 10.1016/j.ccep.2018.05.010

[18] Lustgarten DL, Crespo EM, Arkhipova-Jenkins I, et al. His-bundle pacing versus biventricular pacing in cardiac resynchronization therapy patients: A crossover design comparison. Heart Rhythm. 2015;12(7):1548-1557. DOI: 10.1016/j.hrthm.2015.03.048

[19] Mar PL, Devabhaktuni SR, Dandamudi G. His Bundle Pacing in Heart Failure-Concept and Current Data. Curr Heart Fail Rep. 2019;16(1):47-56. DOI: 10.1007/s11897-019-0423-2

[20] Sharma PS, Dandamudi G, Herweg B, et al. Permanent His-bundle pacing as an alternative to biventricular pacing for cardiac resynchronization therapy: A multicenter experience. Heart Rhythm. 2018;15(3):413-420. DOI: 10.1016/j.hrthm.2017.10.014

[21] Sharma PS, Naperkowski A, Bauch TD, et al. Permanent His Bundle Pacing for Cardiac Resynchronization Therapy in Patients With Heart Failure and Right Bundle Branch Block. Circ Arrhythm Electrophysiol. 2018;11(9):e006613. DOI: 10.1161/CIRCEP.118.006613

[22] Kaufmann R., Rothberger C.J. Beitragezuret stehungsweise extrasystolischer allorhythmien. Zeitschrift Fur Die Gesamte Experimentelle Medizin. 1919. Vol. 9. P. 104-122.

[23] Narula OS. Longitudinal dissociation in the His bundle. Bundle branch block due to asynchronous conduction within the His bundle in man. Circulation. 1977;56(6):996-1006. DOI: 10.1161/01.cir.56.6.996

[24] Dandamudi G, Vijayaraman P. The Complexity of the His Bundle: Understanding Its Anatomy and Physiology through the Lens of the Past and the Present. Pacing Clin Electrophysiol. 2016;39(12):1294-1297. DOI: 10.1111/pace.12925

[25] Kawashima T, Sasaki H. A macroscopic anatomical investigation of atrioventricular bundle locational variation relative to the membranous part of the ventricular septum in elderly human hearts. Surg Radiol Anat. 2005;27(3):206-213. DOI:10.1007/s00276-004-0302-7

[26] Kronborg MB, Mortensen PT, Poulsen SH, Gerdes JC, Jensen HK, Nielsen JC. His or para-His pacing preserves left ventricular function in atrioventricular block: a double-blind, randomized, crossover study. Europace. 2014;16(8):1189-1196. DOI: 10.1093/europace/euu011

[27] Mar PL, Devabhaktuni SR, Dandamudi G. His Bundle Pacing in Heart Failure-Concept and Current Data. Curr Heart Fail Rep. 2019;16(1):47-56. DOI: 10.1007/s11897-019-0423-2

[28] Ajijola OA, Upadhyay GA, Macias C, Shivkumar K, Tung R. Permanent His-bundle pacing for cardiac resynchronization therapy: Initial feasibility study in lieu of left ventricular lead. Heart Rhythm. 2017;14(9):1353-1361. DOI: 10.1016/j.hrthm.2017.04.003

[29] Upadhyay GA, Tung R. His Bundle Pacing for Cardiac Resynchronization. Card Electrophysiol Clin. 2018;10(3):511-517. DOI: 10.1016/j.ccep.2018.05.010

[30] Vijayaraman P, Dandamudi G, Zanon F, et al. Permanent His bundle pacing: Recommendations from a Multicenter His Bundle Pacing Collaborative Working Group for standardization of definitions, implant measurements, and follow-up. Heart Rhythm. 2018;15(3):460-468. DOI: 10.1016/j.hrthm.2017.10.039

[31] Vijayaraman P. His-bundle Pacing to Left Bundle Branch Pacing: Evolution of His-Purkinje Conduction System Pacing. J Innov Card Rhythm Manag. 2019;10(5):3668-3673. Published 2019 May 15. DOI: 10.19102/icrm.2019.100504

[32] Zanon F, Ellenbogen KA, Dandamudi G, et al. Permanent His-bundle pacing: a systematic literature review and meta-analysis. Europace. 2018;20(11):1819-1826. DOI: 10.1093/europace/euy058

[33] Vijayaraman P, Herweg B, Ellenbogen KA, Gajek J. His-Optimized Cardiac Resynchronization Therapy to Maximize Electrical Resynchronization: A Feasibility Study. Circ Arrhythm Electrophysiol. 2019;12(2):e006934. DOI: 10.1161/CIRCEP.118.006934

[34] Lustgarten DL, Crespo EM, Arkhipova-Jenkins I, et al. His-bundle pacing versus biventricular pacing in cardiac resynchronization therapy patients: A crossover design comparison. Heart Rhythm. 2015;12(7):1548-1557. DOI: 10.1016/j.hrthm.2015.03.048

[35] Lustgarten DL. His Bundle Pacing: Getting on the Learning Curve. Card Electrophysiol Clin. 2018;10(3):491-494. DOI: 10.1016/j.ccep.2018.05.012.

[36] Jastrzębski M, Moskal P, Hołda MK, Strona M, Bednarek A, Kiełbasa G, Czarnecka D. Deep septal deployment of a thin, lumenless pacing lead: a translational cadaver simulation study. Europace. 2020 Jan 1;22(1):156-161. DOI: 10.1093/europace/euz270

Chapter 5

Out-of-Hospital Cardiac Arrest in General Population and Sudden Cardiac Death in Athletes

Bettina Nagy, Boldizsár Kiss, Gábor Áron Fülöp and Endre Zima

Abstract

Sudden cardiac death (SCD) is still one of the leading causes of cardiovascular death in the developed countries. The incidence of out-of-hospital cardiac arrest in Europe varies from 67 to 170 per 100,000 population. The chain of survival will be described in detailed steps. We are going to summarize the treatment options for sudden cardiac arrest from recognition of SCD to resuscitation and post cardiac arrest care. The role of awereness and Automated External Defibrillator and Public Access Defibrillation (AED-PAD) programs will be discussed in brief. SCD is one of the most common causes of death among athletes. Sport can trigger SCD in individuals who already have unknown form of heart disease. Our aim was to detail the underlying causes of SCD in athletes and to identify the possible screening techniques. Existing disease (e.g., myocardial hypertrophy, fibrosis) can be seen as a substrate, and sport as a trigger can cause arrhythmias, increased catecholamine release, acidosis, and dehydration. We will highlight the importance of sports medicine and periodic examination in screening for these conditions. Depending on the etiology, this may include exercise ECG, Holter monitor, CT, MR, echocardiography, and coronagraphy. We are going to conclude the new recommendations for COVID-19 post-infection care for athletes.

Keywords: sudden cardiac death, out-of-hospital cardiac arrest, in-hospital cardiac arrest, resuscitation, post cardiac arrest care, COVID-19 infection, athletes

1. Introduction

Despite the advances in diagnosis and treatment during the past decades, sudden cardiac death (SCD) is one of the most common causes of cardiovascular mortality. There are several definitions of SCD in the literature [1]. According to the most widely used one, sudden cardiac death is a set of symptoms in which natural, unexpected death occurs within 1 hour of the onset of symptoms. However, this definition applies only if the death itself has an eyewitness. Failing this, SCD is considered to be the cause of death if the person was still being well, 24 hours before the body was found [2–4].

Based on the location of SCD, one can divide out-of-hospital (OHCA) and in-hospital sudden cardiac arrest (IHCA). Data on adult mortality from sudden cardiac

IntechOpen

death due to cardiovascular disease could not be adequately characterized for a long time. This is mainly due to a lack of well-designed clinical research, inaccurate data collection, and an unclear definition.

Sudden cardiac death is rare among athletes. It is a devastating phenomenon, as athletes are associated with the image of a strong, healthy, resilient body. These cases usually get in focus of media publicity, and even if, for a short time, sudden cardiac death gets the spotlight. This is also of great importance to the public because it draws attention to the importance of expertise in resuscitation.

We are going to point out the importance and process of resuscitation and prevention strategies in this chapter. The role of screening of athletes will be discussed.

2. Incidence of out-of-hospital sudden cardiac death (OHCA)

The epidemiological, clinical, and pathological characteristics of out-of-hospital SCD are inadequately defined for several reasons.

First, in a significant proportion of clinical research studies, OHCA is not detected because it occurs unexpectedly. Death certificates, medical histories, consultations with relatives, and questionnaires completed by them are reliable sources of

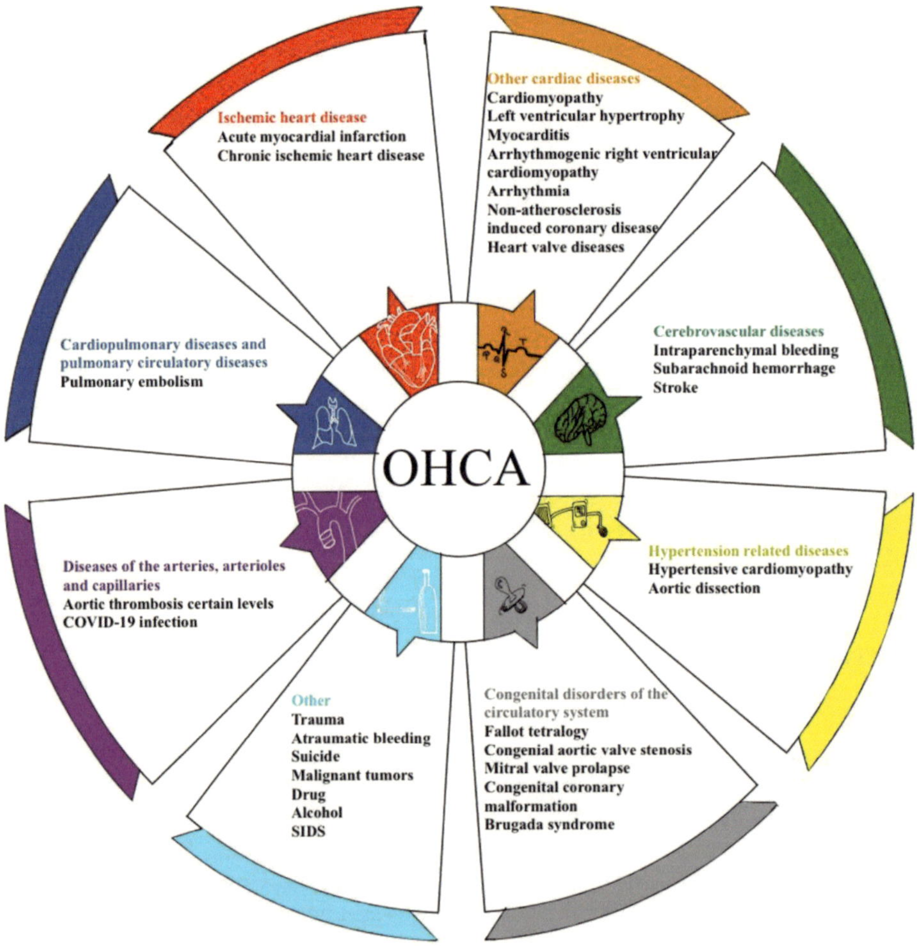

Figure 1.
The most common causes of OHCA (own flowchart).

information but often show uncertainty about the cause of death. Second, very few studies consider autopsy-based data that determine the cause of sudden cardiac arrest. In all cases, a complete autopsy, including a toxicological and histopathological examination, should be performed, to investigate the possibility of sudden cardiac death [5]. On the other hand, causes of death based on death certificates are inaccurate and, as a consequence, overestimate the incidence of sudden cardiac arrest [6, 7]. Third, emergency documentation often does not include cases of SCD outside the hospital without an eyewitness, and sometimes these medical records are not available. Last, different SCD definitions are used in the studies, making them difficult to compare.

The incidence of sudden cardiac deaths is usually estimated from studies in developed countries. Fortunately, we still have some reliable data regarding the incidence. OHCA is recorded in about 70% of European countries, but unfortunately, the data record is not uniform. The European Registry of Cardiac Arrest (EuReCa) involved 29 countries with an annual incidence of OHCA in Europe of between 67 and 170 per 100,000 population [1]. The causes show significant variations by gender and age. Incidence is 3–4 times higher in men than in women and increases with age [8].

2.1 Etiology of OHCA

Ischemic heart disease is the most common cause of out-of-hospital sudden cardiac death. Causes of death also include cardiomyopathy, cerebrovascular disease, and arrhythmia (see **Figure 1**). In contrast, there are cases where the death due to a sudden cardiac arrest occurs outside the hospital, and this is the first appearance of the disease [3, 9, 10].

3. Awareness

Prevention is separated by definition to primary and secondary prevention. In the case of primary prevention, the goal is to screen patients who are at high risk for SCD but have not had SCD in their lifetime and have not had a malignant arrhythmia. Prevention of sudden cardiac death primarily involves the elimination and treatment of cardiovascular risk factors with smoking cessation, increased physical activity, special diet, treatment of high blood pressure, diabetes, high blood fat, and weight loss in case of obesity. Preventive strategies also aim to define groups or individuals at increased risk of SCD in specific populations. Typically, patients with decreased left ventricular ejection fraction are at high risk for SCD, but a cardiovascular risk assessment of competitive athletes would also be essential.

During secondary prevention, the goal is to further treat patients who have successfully resuscitated after SCD or who have had a malignant arrhythmia and to prevent another arrhythmia.

4. Treatment of circulatory arrest: resuscitation

The formal professional opinion on resuscitation is published every 5 years by the European Resuscitation Council (ERC) in the form of a recommendation, following the scientific preparation of the International Liaison Committee on Resuscitation (ILCOR). The ERC Directive 2021, published this year, is currently in force [11].

According to the terminology of the ILCOR Consensus on Science with Treatment Recommendations (CoSTR), resuscitation should be initiated in any person who is "unresponsive and absent or abnormal in breathing [12]. This terminology is also included in the most recent basic life support (BLS) directive 2021 [11].

4.1 Basic life support (BLS)

In Hungary, the average arrival of an ambulance is 5–8 minutes, and the first shock is delivered 8–11 minutes after the announcement [13]. During this time, the survival of the patient is in the hands of the layman. The use of BLS and the use of an automated external defibrillator (AED) can significantly improve long-term survival.

Patient survival is determined by elements of the chain of survival from circulatory arrest. It includes early recognition of cardiac arrest and calling for help, circulatory maintenance with high-quality chest compression and rescue breathing, early defibrillation (if necessary), and post-cardiac arrest intensive care after achieving return of spontaneous circulation (ROSC) (**Figure 2**).

The survival chain shown in the figure symbolizes the steps required to perform the circulatory arrest. The first three steps on site can be done by anyone. Abbreviations: AED: Automated External Defibrillator.

4.1.1 How to recognize a sudden cardiac arrest?

- Any person who does not respond and breathing is absent or is abnormal, one should consider that the patient is in cardiac arrest. CPR should be started immediately.

- Slow, agonal breathing should be considered a sign of sudden cardiac arrest, as in almost 40% of cases, this symptom occurs immediately after circulatory arrest.

- Short-term, seizure activity may occur at the onset of cardiac arrest, the person should be examined after the termination of the seizure: if he does not respond and is short of breath or abnormal, CPR should be started.

4.1.2 What to do in case of sudden cardiac arrest?

How to call for help?

- The National Ambulance Service must be notified immediately for resuscitation.

- If the eyewitness is alone and has a mobile phone after the emergency call, one should turn on the speaker of the phone and start CPR immediately.

- If the eyewitness is alone and does not have a cell phone, the patient should first be left there until he or she notifies the ambulance service, and then CPR should begin as soon as possible.

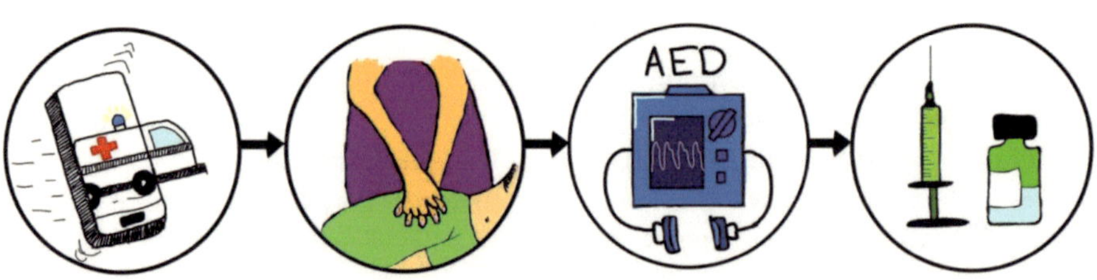

Figure 2.
The survival chain (own flowchart).

How to perform quality chest compression?

- Compression should be performed on the lower half of the patient's sternum.
- Depth can be approximately 5 cm, but not more than 6 cm.
- Its frequency is 100–120 compression/minute.
- Full chest release is required, do not lean on the chest.
- If possible, it should be performed on a patient lying on a hard surface.

How to perform rescue breath?

- After 30 chest compressions, two rescue breaths are to be given.
- If rescue breathing is not possible, chest compression must be continued without interruption.
- In case of risk of infection (for example: during the COVID-19 epidemic), continuous chest compression is required until professional help is obtained, without rescue breathing.

4.1.3 AED-PAD program

Local-regional AED-PAD (automated external defibrillator–public access defibrillation) programs are essential to reduce time till return of spontaneous circulation, the central nervous system ischemic injury, and to improve survival. In the case of a shockable rhythm, defibrillation within 3–5 minutes of collapse can result in survival of up to 50–70% [13–15]. Delaying defibrillation reduces survival by approximately 10–12% per minute. AEDs are easy to use, but proper training is required to master them properly. The PAD program aims to reduce the number of deaths due to sudden cardiac arrest in public places. The AED is to be located in high-traffic areas that are accessible to all, e.g., airports, stadiums, schools, shopping malls. It helps laypeople with simple voice instructions during resuscitation. Based on a defined algorithm, it performs a rhythm analysis every 2 minutes and, if it detects a rhythm to be shocked, charges the defibrillation capacitor, and then the resuscitator can deliver the shock with the push of a highlighted button.

4.2 Advanced life support (ALS)

The ERC guidelines are based on the 2020 ILCOR CoSTR. There have been no significant changes to the 2021 adult ALS guidelines [11]. Priority remains on high-quality chest compression with minimal interruption and early defibrillation. Chest compression should be paused only when necessary, for as short a time as possible, in the event of a shock, care should be taken not exceeding 5 seconds. The use of airway management devices must comply with the principle of gradation, i.e., from the simplest to the more complex. There has also been no change in resuscitation drugs. In the case of a non-shockable rhythm, 1 mg of adrenaline should be used as soon as possible, and in the case of a shockable rhythm, an additional 1 mg of adrenaline should be given every 3–5 minutes after the third shock and until the return of spontaneous circulation. If the shockable rhythm cannot be terminated, an iv. bolus of 300 mg amiodarone after the third shock, an additional iv. bolus of

150 mg amiodarone should be given after the fifth shock. During the advanced life support, the aim is to clarify reversible causes according to 4H/4 T: hypoxia, hypo-hyperkalemia, hypovolemia, hypothermia, thromboembolism (coronary, pulmonary), toxin, tamponade, tension pneumothorax. The new guideline recognizes the growing role of bedside point-of-care ultrasound (POCUS) in clarifying the etiology, but stresses the need for a competent handler and to minimize interruptions during chest compression associated with the use of POCUS. The guidelines also reflect the consideration of increasingly evidence-based extracorporeal techniques (eCPR) as rescue therapy to facilitate ALS failure and to facilitate certain interventions (coronary angiography, percutaneous coronary intervention, pulmonary thrombectomy).

5. Post-cardiac arrest syndrome (PCAS)

In 2015, the ERC and the European Society of Intensive Care Medicine developed the first combined resuscitation treatment guidelines, which were jointly published in Resuscitation and Intensive Care Medicine [16]. The latest version, published in 2021, including the directive with new results since 2015, supplemented by further recommendations [17].

In post-resuscitation care, ensuring adequate oxygenation, ventilation, and circulating cardiac output remain one of the cornerstones of care, and cerebral protection is paramount. The Recommendation describes the four key components of the PCAS to be focused on during early treatment that are still accepted today. These include post-circulatory central nervous system damage, post-circulatory myocardial dysfunction, systemic ischemic and reperfusion responses, and persistent underlying disease-causing circulatory arrest.

If the patient's spontaneous circulation has returned, treatment of PCAS is initiated on-site, with the pillars of stabilization of the hemodynamic state, prevention of arrhythmia recurrence, prevention of cellular damage, and normalization of organ perfusion. Following on-site stabilization, patient care will be continued in specialized centers capable of providing full diagnostic and therapeutic care, which will include a high-level intensive care, angiography, and electrophysiology laboratory, CT/MRI, neurology, mechanical circulatory support, and cardiac surgery.

One of the most important elements of intensive PCAS treatment is controlled targeted temperature management, which is essential to prevent hypoxic and further secondary damage to the brain. Neurological damage is exacerbated during hyperpyrexia, epileptiform seizure activities, and hypoglycemia during PCAS [6]. The quality of treatment applied in the early post-resuscitation period significantly determines the outcome, especially concerning neurological recovery [18].

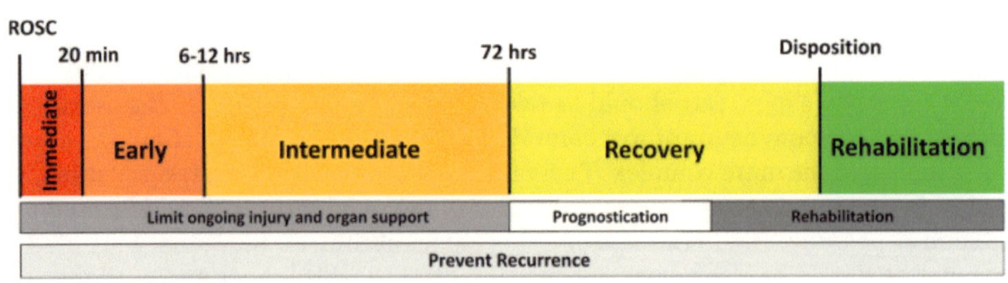

Figure 3.
Phases of return of spontaneous circulation (ROSC) [19].

The consecutive phases of PCAS and the intervals of care are illustrated in **Figure 3**. Time intervals may vary from patient to patient after the first 20 minutes after a spontaneous return of circulation (ROSC), depending on the severity of the PCAS, the rate of recovery, or any progression that may occur. At each stage, care is aimed at limiting ongoing injuries and preventing recurrence of cardiac arrest.

1. Immediate phase: The first 20 minutes after ROSC, part of primary care and delivery to a designated health care facility, stabilization.

2. Early phase: The period between 20 minutes and 6–12 hours after ROSC. Early interventions (causal treatment and initiation of therapeutic hypothermia) may be most effective here.

3. Transitional phase: 12–72 hours, the injury mechanisms are still active, usually aggressive treatment is required.

4. Recovery phase: from about 72 hours to the 7th day. The onset may vary from patient to patient, the timing being influenced by cardiovascular status or the use of therapeutic hypothermia. The prognosis estimation is already reliable at this stage.

5. The rehabilitation phase.

6. Sudden cardiac death in athletes

Sudden cardiac death is rare among athletes, but it is still a devastating phenomenon, as athletes are associated with the image of a strong, healthy, resilient body. These cases usually get into the focus of media attention, and even if, for a short time, SCD gets in the spotlight. This is also of great importance to the public because it draws attention to having expertise in resuscitation.

The likelihood of OHCA in athletes is also influenced by age, gender, the type of sport, and the existing diseases. The incidence is between 1/50,000 and 1/100,000 in young athletes on an annual basis [20]. An athlete is considered to be young under the age 35. Among them, SCD is usually a consequence of some congenital disease. The incidence rises between 1/15,000 and 1/18,000 in elderly athletes [21]. In these cases, sudden cardiac death is usually associated with coronary disease [20]. Similar to the general population, male athletes have a higher risk of SCD compared with their female counterparts (5:1) [21].

The type of sport and the intensity of the activity performed are also influencing factors. Observations suggest that basketball, football, and athletics have the highest risk of SCD [21]. Hobby athletes who have congenital disorders should choose a sport that can be pursued at a constant energy level, avoiding a sudden increase in the heart rate. In addition, it is also worth avoiding extreme environment during sports, such as high temperature and high humidity. These can adversely affect blood pressure and electrolyte balance [20].

In some cases, the underlying cardiovascular disease in athletes remains asymptomatic, and the first symptom is sudden cardiac arrest. Although in the minority of the cases, syncope, chest pain, and ventricular arrhythmias appear as warning symptoms.

Cardiac and non-cardiac diseases leading to sudden cardiac death in athletes, grouped by age, are listed in **Table 1**.

Causes of SCD (under 35 years)	Causes of SCD (over 35 years)
Hypertrophic cardiomyopathy	Coronary disease
Arrhythmogenic right ventricular cardiomyopathy	Aortic dissection
Coronary heart disease	Pulmonary embolism
Aortic aneurysm	Ischemic heart disease
Myocarditis	
Ion channel mutation	
Ruptured aortic aneurysm	
Heart valve disease	
Congenital heart disease	

Table 1.
Causes of SCD based on age.

6.1 Etiology

Hypertrophic cardiomyopathy is a genetic disorder associated with left ventricular hypertrophy that can lead to SCD via ventricular tachycardia/fibrillation. Basso et al. have found that in athletes, arrhythmogenic right ventricular cardiomyopathy (ARVD) causes sudden cardiac arrest even more often than hypertrophic cardiomyopathy. This genetic disease causes a fatty-fibrous remodeling of the right ventricular wall muscle, and sometimes it affects the left ventricle or the interventricular system as well, which can lead to the aneurysm-like dilation of the ventricular free wall [22].

Congenital coronary abnormalities may also be in the background of sudden cardiac death. According to one study, these are responsible for 17% of athletes' deaths from cardiovascular disease. One of the most severe coronary malformations is the origin of the coronary artery from behind the pulmonary trunk, which causes severe symptoms from an early age. However, other lesions with less pronounced symptoms can also cause SCD, especially during increased exercise. In these cases, the coronary can be derived from the sinus on the opposite side, which will make its course abnormal. During exercise, an abnormally grown coronary artery cannot increase blood flow sufficiently, leading to the development of ischemic episodes. As a result, the myocardium will be injured, and the resulting scar tissue will serve as a basis for ventricular arrhythmias and ventricular fibrillation [23].

Pathologists do not find any myocardial lesion that causes SCD in 30% of autopsies. In such cases, cardiac arrest may have been caused by ion channel mutations (long QT syndrome, Brugada syndrome), which may eventually result in ventricular fibrillation. Mutation of ion channels may be alerted by ECG abnormality. The disease is inherited by autosomal dominant, and the mutation is found in genes encoding sodium and potassium channels. Catecholaminergic polymorphic ventricular tachycardia can develop due to a mutation in calcium receptors. In this case, we do not see any difference in the resting ECG. However, with increased sympathetic activity during sports activities, arrhythmias may occur above a heart rate of 120–130/min [22].

Among the valve defects, mitral valve prolapse and aortic stenosis, which are arrhythmogenic, should be highlighted. The most common cause of aortic stenosis is calcareous disease of the aortic valve, with manifestation at a much younger age in addition to bicuspid aortic valves [22].

Acquired cardiac abnormalities may also be among the underlying causes, such as myocarditis due to a viral infection, vascular disease, and aortic dissection [23].

6.2 Why is screening important?

Sport activity can trigger sudden cardiac death in individuals who already have some kind of heart disease. Existing disease (e.g., hypertrophy, fibrosis) can be considered as a substrate and sport may be a trigger, which can cause arrhythmias, increased catecholamine release, acidosis, and dehydration [23].

The American Heart Association and the Sports Cardiology Study Group of the European Society of Cardiology recommend physical examination of high school and college students before a sporting activity in addition to their own and family history recordings. The European guidelines complement this with an ECG registration. The effectiveness of this screening method is supported by observation published by Corrado et al.; they found that the incidence of sudden cardiac death between 1979 and 1980 decreased from 3.6 athletes/100,000 people/year to 0.4 athletes/100,000 people/year for the year 2004 due to the introduction of screening.

7. COVID-19 and sports

In our experience to date, COVID-19 can damage heart itself and its function in at least two basic ways. Directly, when the virus enters the body by binding to human ACE-2 receptors, which are expressed not only in the lungs but also in the myocardium and several other areas of the cardiovascular system. In the early stages of COVID-associated myocarditis, the virus replicates within myocytes, followed by a subacute immunological response including both the T-cell and B-cell immune responses. At this time, the host's immune system may even worsen myocardial damage through cytokine activation and the production of antibodies to viral proteins. In the chronic phase of myocarditis, fibrosis and dilatation of the ventricles may occur. This may manifest as deterioration in pump function and may lead to heart failure [24]. According to a study presented by Linder et al. [25], the presence of Sars-Cov-2 in the myocardium (24/39 autopsy pattern, 61.5%) and active viral replication suggested that direct viral invasion may be more common than previously it was previously assumed. In these studies, the samples were taken from patients treated in hospitals; therefore, their applicability to athletes in the younger population has not been established. The other way in which an intense "cytokine storm" during a severe disease leads to a decrease in heart function, similarly to other forms of sepsis, with mechanisms that are overlapping the development of "stress" or catecholamine-induced cardiomyopathy [25].

Although hospitalization for acute infection in young, healthy individuals is uncommon, there is concern that subclinical myocardial damage may be present in several cases and may manifest as prolonged malaise, or even more may develop malignant arrhythmias and may act as substrate for cardiac death. Exercise during the acute phase of myocarditis caused by a viral infection can accelerate or prolong the disease and trigger malignant and nonmalignant arrhythmias (**Figure 4**) [20].

Therefore, it is important to emphasize that training started before the recommended recovery period of time may contribute to involve cardiovascular system even in asymptomatic individuals. Athletes must undergo a full cardiological examination before returning to daily training. Transthoracic echocardiography is currently considered the first line in post-COVID-19 monitoring in athletes. In addition, exercise ECG and 24-hour Holter monitoring are also a useful help in the "return-to-play" algorithm to detect possible supraventricular and ventricular arrhythmias but have low sensitivity to identify myocarditis [26]. Finally, the levels of serum biomarkers (troponin, CK-MB, BNP) should be monitored thoroughly.

Athletes having positive COVID 19 test or experienced symptoms should abstain from sports and strenuous physical activity for 2 weeks. In the case of myocarditis

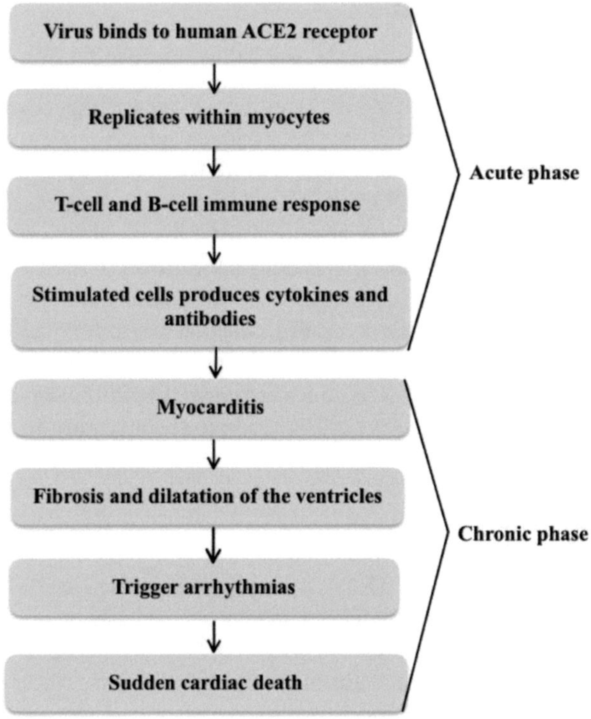

Figure 4.
COVID-19 disease progression in the heart.

or myopericarditis, athletes need to be withheld in sport activity for up to 3–6 months depending on the course and severity of the disease [27]. Thereafter, if the left ventricular systolic function has returned to normal, serum biomarkers for myocardial damage started to decrease, and no clinically significant supraventricular or ventricular arrhythmia has been observed in the 24-hour Holter monitoring or during exercise test, the athlete can return to sport activity [28].

8. Summary

More than half of cardiovascular deaths in the 35–49-year-old population are out-of-hospital non-traumatic sudden cardiac arrest. The rate, for men, is 3–4 times higher than for women; and it gradually increases with age. The classical cardiovascular risk factors are obesity, hypertension, diabetes mellitus, hyperlipidemia, and smoking, in addition to cardiac morphology as known coronary disease or cardiac myopathies can cause sudden cardiac death.

Regular screening significantly reduced the incidence of sudden cardiac death among athletes as well.

A growing number of studies suggest that many COVID-19 survivors experience some type of heart damage, including arrhythmias, heart failure, and myocarditis, even if they were asymptomatic. Congenital structural diseases and myocarditis are a leading cause of sudden cardiac death in competitive athletes so they must be properly treated by their cardiologists before the return to sports.

Exponentially increasing number of scientific data on OHCA and IHCA are available to help with prevention as well. Future studies processing histopathological and toxicological data from autopsy may provide adequate medical data to develop a strategy to prevent cardiovascular death.

Author details

Bettina Nagy, Boldizsár Kiss, Gábor Áron Fülöp and Endre Zima*
Heart and Vascular Center, Semmelweis University, Budapest, Hungary

*Address all correspondence to: zima.endre@gmail.com

References

[1] Perkins GD et al. European Resuscitation Council Guidelines 2021: Executive summary. Resuscitation. 2021;**161**:1-60

[2] Priori SG et al. 2015 ESC Guidelines for the management of patients with ventricular arrhythmias and the prevention of sudden cardiac death: The Task Force for the Management of Patients with Ventricular Arrhythmias and the Prevention of Sudden Cardiac Death of the European Society of Cardiology (ESC) Endorsed by: Association for European Paediatric and Congenital Cardiology (AEPC). European Heart Journal. 2015;**36**:2793-2867

[3] Tubaro M, Vranckx P, Price S, Vrints C. The ESC Textbook of Intensive and Acute Cardiovascular Care. The European Society of Cardiology: Oxford University Press; 2015. DOI: 10.1093/med/9780199687039.001.0001 [Published online on Feb 2018]

[4] Moore MJ et al. Demographic and temporal trends in out of hospital sudden cardiac death in Belfast. Heart (British Cardiac Society). 2006;**92**:311-315

[5] Gorgels APM, Gijsbers C, de Vreede-Swagemakers J, Lousberg A, Wellens HJJ. Out-of-hospital cardiac arrest-the relevance of heart failure. The Maastricht Circulatory Arrest Registry. European Heart Journal. 2003;**24**:1204-1209

[6] Filippi A et al. Out of hospital sudden cardiac death in Italy: A population-based case–control study. Journal of Cardiovascular Medicine. 2008;**9**: 595-600

[7] Kannel WB, Cupples LA, D'Agostino RB. Sudden death risk in overt coronary heart disease: The Framingham Study. American Heart Journal. 1987;**113**:799-804

[8] Morentin B, Audicana C. Population-based study of out-of-hospital sudden cardiovascular death: Incidence and causes of death in middle-aged adults. Revista Española de Cardiología (English Edition). 2011;**64**:28-34

[9] Chugh SS et al. Current burden of sudden cardiac death: Multiple source surveillance versus retrospective death certificate-based review in a large U.S. community. Journal of the American College of Cardiology. 2004;**44**:1268-1275

[10] Byrne R et al. Multiple source surveillance incidence and aetiology of out-of-hospital sudden cardiac death in a rural population in the West of Ireland. European Heart Journal. 2008;**29**:1418-1423

[11] Semeraro F et al. European Resuscitation Council guidelines 2021: Systems saving lives. Resuscitation. 2021;**161**:80-97

[12] Koster RW et al. European Resuscitation Council guidelines for Resuscitation 2010 section 2. Adult basic life support and use of automated external defibrillators. Resuscitation. 2010;**81**:1277-1292

[13] Gobl G, Gaspar T. Out-of-hospital cardiac arrest in Hungary: The Utstein database. Resuscitation. 2006;**70**:308

[14] Valenzuela TD et al. Outcomes of rapid defibrillation by security officers after cardiac arrest in casinos. New England Journal of Medicine. 2000;**343**:1206-1209

[15] Berdowski J et al. Impact of onsite or dispatched automated external defibrillator use on survival after out-of-hospital cardiac arrest. Circulation. 2011;**124**:2225-2232

[16] Nolan JP et al. European Resuscitation Council and European

Society of Intensive Care Medicine Guidelines for Post-resuscitation Care 2015: Section 5 of the European Resuscitation Council Guidelines for Resuscitation 2015. Resuscitation. 2015;**95**:202-222

[17] Nolan JP et al. European Resuscitation Council and European Society of Intensive Care Medicine guidelines 2021: Post-resuscitation care. Intensive Care Medicine. 2021;**47**:369-421

[18] Søholm H et al. Tertiary centres have improved survival compared to other hospitals in the Copenhagen area after out-of-hospital cardiac arrest. Resuscitation. 2013;**84**:162-167

[19] Topjian AA et al. Pediatric post–cardiac arrest care: A scientific statement from the American Heart Association. Circulation. 2019;**140**:e194-e233

[20] Pelliccia A et al. Recommendations for participation in competitive and leisure time sport in athletes with cardiomyopathies, myocarditis, and pericarditis: Position statement of the Sport Cardiology Section of the European Association of Preventive Cardiology (EAPC). European Heart Journal. 2019;**40**:19-33

[21] Lorvidhaya P, Stephen Huang SK. Sudden cardiac death in athletes. Cardiology. 2003;**100**:186-195

[22] Basso C, Rizzo S, Carturan E, Pilichou K, Thiene G. Cardiac arrest at rest and during sport activity: Causes and prevention. European Heart Journal Supplements: Journal of the European Society of Cardiology. 2020;**22**:E20-E24

[23] Semsarian C, Sweeting J, Ackerman MJ. Sudden cardiac death in athletes. British Journal of Sports Medicine. 2015;**49**:1017

[24] Lindner D et al. Association of cardiac infection with SARS-CoV-2 in confirmed COVID-19 autopsy cases. JAMA Cardiology. 2020;**5**:1281-1285

[25] Clerkin KJ et al. COVID-19 and cardiovascular disease. Circulation. 2020;**141**:1648-1655

[26] Phelan D et al. Screening of potential cardiac involvement in competitive athletes recovering from COVID-19: An expert consensus statement. JACC: Cardiovascular Imaging. 2020;**13**:2635-2652

[27] Hurwitz B, Issa O. Management and treatment of myocarditis in athletes. Current Treatment Options in Cardiovascular Medicine. 2020;**22**:65

[28] Dores H, Cardim N. Return to play after COVID-19: A sport cardiologist's view. British Journal of Sports Medicine. 2020;**54**:1132

Chapter 6

Life-Threatening Cardiac Arrhythmias during Anesthesia and Surgery

Zuraini Md. Noor

Abstract

Life-threatening arrhythmias are frequently encountered during anesthesia for cardiac or non-cardiac surgery. They result in a significant cause of morbidity and mortality, particularly in elderly patients. Predisposing factors like electrolytes abnormalities, pre-existing cardiac disease, intubation procedure, anesthetic medications, and various surgical stimulation need to be determined. Early diagnosis and commencement of an appropriate treatment protocol may be lifesaving. Treatment usually involves correction of the underlying causes, cardiac electroversion, and the use of one or more antiarrhythmic agents. Although ventricular tachycardia, ventricular fibrillation, torsade de pointes, and pulseless electrical activity are considered malignant arrhythmias that can lead to cardiac arrest, other types of Brady and tachyarrhythmias are also included in this chapter to enable adopting a more objective approach in the management of arrhythmias intraoperatively, avoiding risks of inappropriate management strategies.

Keywords: arrhythmias, anesthesia, surgery, life-threatening, intraoperatively

1. Introduction

1.1 Definition of cardiac arrhythmias

Accelerated, slowed, or irregular heart rates caused by abnormalities in the electrical impulses of the myocardium.

Cardiac arrhythmias are very common in the general population and are a significant cause of morbidity and mortality of both cardiac and noncardiac surgical procedures during the perioperative period. While the incidence of perioperative arrhythmias is extremely high (the Multicenter Study of General Anesthesia reported a 70.2% incidence of Brady and tachyarrhythmias in 17,201 patients having general anesthesia for a variety of surgical procedures), only 1.6% of these required clinically significant management [1–3]. For cardiac surgery, the patients are more prone to develop arrhythmias with a reported incidence of greater than 90%, while incidence for patients undergoing non-cardiac surgery is lower and varies from 16.3 to 61.7% [4–6]. Patients with pre-existing cardiac disease for cardiac surgery are more prone to develop perioperative rhythm disturbances. It is obvious that arrhythmias that occur during surgery are clinically important as it can evolve to life-threatening malignant arrhythmias with severe hemodynamic instability and

Class	Actions	Drugs (examples)
I	Sodium channel blockade	
IA	~moderate	Quinidine, procainamide
IB	~weak	Lidocaine, mexiletine
IC	~strong	Flecainide, propafenone
II	β blockade	Propranolol, esmolol, sotalol
III	Potassium (K^+) channel blocker	Amiodarone, ibutilide
IV	Calcium (Ca^{2+}) channel blocker	Diltiazem, verapamil

Table 1.
Choice of antiarrhythmic therapies based on Vaughan-Williams classification (classes I–IV).

cardiovascular collapse, necessitating prompt initiation of adequate cardiopulmonary resuscitation (CPR) and defibrillation or electrical cardioversion. Hence, a thorough understanding and prompt diagnosis and intervention are critical for the anesthesiologist in order to reduce severe perioperative adverse outcomes.

An understanding of normal cardiac physiology is essential before rhythm disturbances can be understood. The normal cardiac electrical conduction system is responsible for the contraction of the heart muscle and is represented on the electrocardiogram.

Normal cardiac conduction begins with cardiac impulses coming from the sinoatrial node and travels to both atria. The atria depolarizes and generates the P wave. From here, the impulse propagates to the atrioventricular node, then reaches the his bundle and Purkinje fibers transforming into conduction, causing ventricular contraction and generates the QRS wave [6]. The resting sinus heart rate in adults is usually between 60 and 100 beats/min.

In the heart, electrical stimulation is created by a sequence of ion fluxes through specialized channels in the cardiomyocytes that generate action potential and lead to a coordinated cardiac contraction in systole. Each action potential corresponds to one beat of the heart and the inherent frequency of these cells is essential for maintaining proper rate control. Antiarrhythmic drugs act by modifying this action potential, which results from the alteration of ion channels (**Table 1**).

Five phases of cardiac action potential (as illustrated in **Figure 1**):

- Phase 4: resting potential at –90 mV with minor depolarization from –90 mV to –70 mV; the passive outflow of potassium.
- Phase 0: rapid depolarization from –70 mV to +50 mV; inward voltage-gated sodium channels.
- Phase 1: minor repolarization; outward voltage-gated potassium channels.
- Phase 2: plateau at +50 mV; outward voltage-gated potassium channels and inward voltage-gated calcium channels.
- Phase 3: repolarization from +50 mV to –90 mV; outward voltage-gated potassium channels.

Damage to the normal conduction system of the heart can lead to rhythm disturbances which can be either benign or more serious in nature depending on the hemodynamic consequence of the arrhythmia and the possibility of evolving into a lethal arrhythmia.

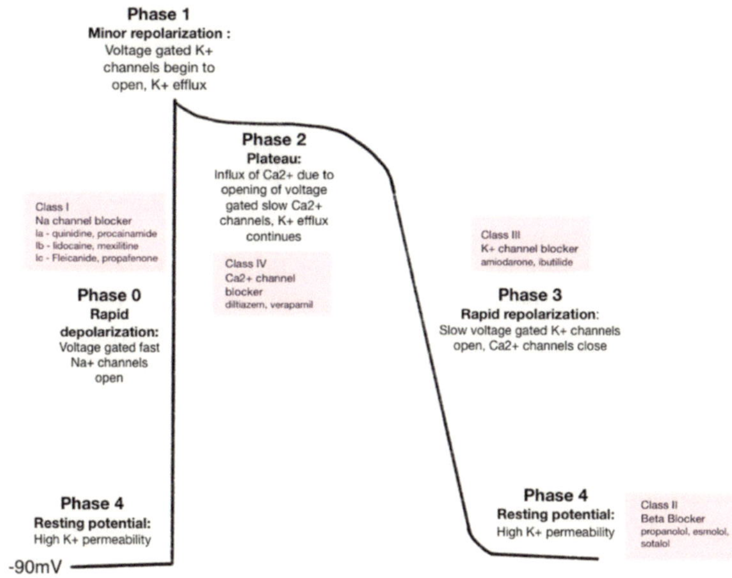

Figure 1.
Cardiac action potential.

Bradyarrhythmias result from decreased intrinsic pacemaker function or blocks in conduction, principally within the AV-node or the His-Purkinje system. Most tachyarrhythmias are caused by re-entry, some result from enhanced normal automaticity or from abnormal mechanisms of automaticity.

2. Mechanism of intraoperative arrhythmias

The principal mechanisms of Brady and tachyarrhythmias which are observed in clinical practice are as follows [5]:

1. Injury to the cardiac conduction system.

2. Re-entry: a mechanism that may precipitate a wide variety of supraventricular and ventricular arrhythmias, implying the presence of a pathologic circuit of an electrical impulse around a functional or anatomic loop.

3. Automaticity: Abnormal depolarization of atrial or ventricular muscle cells during periods of the action potential can lead to arrhythmias.

4. Mutations in ion channels.

5. Ectopic foci.

3. Contributing factors and causes of arrhythmias during anesthesia for surgery

Although the incidence of intraoperative arrhythmias is extremely high, the majority of such arrhythmias are benign and self-limiting. They require no emergency treatment and respond well to pharmacologic interventions or both.

However, in certain patients, some arrhythmias may pose an immediate threat to life by causing profound hemodynamic instability and require urgent clinical attention.

There are several factors likely to contribute to the generation of intraoperative arrhythmias, which can be classified according to patient, anesthesia, and procedures (**Table 2**) [5, 7]. Identifying the causes mainly responsible for intraoperative arrhythmias is prudent before instituting specific therapy or intervention.

Patients with pre-existing heart disease (e.g., myocardial ischemia) have a much higher incidence of arrhythmias intraoperatively. Intracranial pathology such as subarachnoid hemorrhage and raised intracranial pressure can result in ECG abnormalities because of stimulation of the autonomic nervous system.

Airway manipulation most often associated with hemodynamic disturbances is a well-described cause of intraoperative arrhythmias [4, 7, 8]. During anesthesia, arrhythmias can be produced in the presence of a variety of triggering agents and clinical situations such as light plane of anesthesia with hypertension and tachycardia, hypoxemia, and hypercarbia.

Vital organs, such as the brain, heart, and kidneys, must be perfused adequately during general anesthesia and surgery. Most of the anesthetic agents have direct myocardial depressant effects which result in reduced cardiac contractility and sympathetic stimulation of the peripheral vasculature. The net effect is a fall in cardiac output with a fall in perfusing pressure of vital organs secondary to vascular vasodilation. Conversely, tachycardia can have detrimental effects in patients susceptible to ischemia due to reduced myocardial filling time. Even relatively minor fluctuations in cardiovascular and hemodynamic parameters due to arrhythmias can have a significant incidence of various complications, including

Patient-related	Anesthesia related	Surgical related
Pre-existing cardiac disease, thyrotoxicosis, central nervous system disease (e.g., subarachnoid hemorrhage)	Direct laryngoscopy and intubation	Cardiac surgery (intracardiac surgical manipulation)
	Insufficient level of anesthesia	Surgical manipulation during non-cardiac surgery (e.g., traction to the intestine, oculocardiac reflex). Neurosurgical causes, dental surgery, and laparoscopic surgery
Elderly	Local anesthesia (central neuraxial blockade is associated with pharmacological sympathectomy)	
	Mechanical irritation (e.g., central venous lines, pulmonary artery catheter, chest tube)	
	4Hs 4Ts Hypovolemia, hypoxemia, hyper/hypokalemia (electrolyte disorders) and metabolic disorders (acidosis), hypothermia/hyperthermia Tension pneumothorax, tamponade, toxins/drugs, thromboembolism (pulmonary/cardiac)	

Table 2.
Contributing factors and causes of intraoperative arrhythmias.

cardiovascular events, renal failure, infection, and cerebral infarction, particularly among the elderly co-morbid patients undergoing elective and emergency surgery. The use of halothane during induction in children as well as maintenance of anesthesia has been largely superseded by sevoflurane, which is safer. Electrolyte imbalances, abnormal blood gases, and direct cardiac stimulation via catheters influence the occurrence of arrhythmia and conduction abnormalities. The anesthesiologists should be aware of all the drugs used and able to manage the consequences accordingly [8, 9].

Surgical manipulation and cardiopulmonary bypass during cardiac surgery may precipitate arrhythmias. Vagal stimulation in surgical procedures such as during carotid surgery and peritoneal traction produces bradycardia, conduction block, or even asystole. Dental surgery causes profound stimulation of the autonomic nervous system. Thoracic surgery is associated with an incidence of atrial fibrillation.

4. Anesthetic agents and adjuvants related to arrhythmias

Prolonged cardiac repolarization (represented as QT interval on ECG) induced by various anesthetic agents and adjuvant drugs may trigger the appearance of torsade de pointes (TdP), which in some patients degenerate towards malignant ventricular arrhythmias and sudden cardiac arrest [6, 7, 10]. The duration of QT interval, QT corrected for heart rate (QTc), JT interval, QT dispersion (QTd), QT variability index, and transmular dispersion of repolarization (TDR) are the commonly used ECG markers to check for the possibility of various degrees of TdP under different conditions [11]. All volatile anesthetics, especially isoflurane and desflurane cause QT_C prolongation, while sevoflurane demonstrated no effects on TDR. Propofol is generally considered to be non-torsadogenic. The sympathomimetic properties of ketamine may promote the incidents of TdP [11]. Most opioids have no effect on QTc when used at clinically relevant doses. Succinylcholine has been shown to increase QTc, especially when used in conjunction with thiopental while most nondepolarizing muscle relaxants have no effect on the QT interval. Sugammadex at therapeutic doses has no effect on QTc whereas anticholinesterase-anticholinergic antagonism of neuromuscular blockade with neostigmine and glycopyrrolate or atropine causes clinically significant QTc prolongation. The commonly used local anesthetic agents are relatively safe; nevertheless, extensive central neuraxial blocks may increase the duration of QTc. Several antiemetic drugs, such as droperidol, domperidone, and most 5-HT3 antagonists, produce a significant prolongation of QT. The FDA's black box warning of fatal arrhythmias associated with the administration of droperidol leads to a decrease in the use of this medication in recent years. Midazolam seems to have no effect on QTc and TDR. Although dexmedetomidine may cause mild prolongation of QT interval, it is unlikely to cause TdP. It should also be prudent to use dexmedetomidine with caution, especially in patients with bradyarrhythmias tendencies where the risk of QT prolongation is increased [12–15].

5. Diagnostic evaluation

During surgery, it is not always possible to get 12-lead ECG done. The anesthesiologists would have to make the diagnosis by looking at the continuous ECG monitor in the operating room. Changing the sweep speed on the ECG monitor (from 50 to 25 mm/s) may help with the identification of arrhythmias and their management. Lead II and V5 are superior for arrhythmia detection and diagnosis. All available leads are displayed on the intraoperative monitor if arrhythmia develops and cannot be readily diagnosed. For non-cardiac surgery, 12-lead ECG can be obtained as soon as feasible [9, 16].

The blood pressure, arterial oxygen saturation, and temperature also need to be monitored. More advanced monitoring such as invasive arterial pressure, pulmonary artery catheterization, and transoesophageal echocardiography can provide additional clues when assessing the patient for causes of cardiovascular collapse. End-tidal carbon dioxide may help with the effectiveness of chest compressions during cardiopulmonary resuscitation. Estimation of serum electrolytes for verification of renal function is important in patients on medications for arrhythmias.

Adequate precautions should be taken during surgery to prevent the development of intraoperative arrhythmias:

- Surgical manipulations which can precipitate arrhythmias should be kept to a minimum.

- Adequate depth of anesthesia may prevent or control intraoperative arrhythmias.

- Hypoxia, hypotension, hypovolemia, hypothermia should be prevented during surgery.

Whenever an arrhythmia develops in the intraoperative period, the anesthesiologists should first be able to eliminate the possible causes of arrhythmia before instituting specific interventions. Attempts to correct them should be made while continuing to evaluate the arrhythmia.

6. Specific intra-operative arrhythmias

6.1 Antiarrhythmic drugs

Patients requiring oral antiarrhythmic should continue the medication until the time of surgery. Specific cardiologist consultation is advised for patients who require pacing-cardioverter devices to suppress or terminate tachyarrhythmias. With life-threatening circulatory compromise, prompt pacing or electroversion is required. Obvious electrolyte imbalance should be corrected, and management provided for underlying heart disease. Specific antiarrhythmic agents are used to suppress arrhythmias and prevent recurrences (**Table 3**).

The administration of antiarrhythmic drugs may paradoxically aggravate the arrhythmias that are being treated or cause new rhythm disorders. This is known as proarrhythmia generally occurs when the dosage of drugs does not exceed the therapeutic range [17]. Proarrhythmia is now considered omnipresent with all antiarrhythmic medications. Care should be taken when using antiarrhythmic drugs in patients with structural heart disease, as they are at higher risk of proarrhythmia with antiarrhythmic medications. These patients, such as heart failure or cardiomyopathy are not candidates for Class IC or Class III antiarrhythmics other than amiodarone or sotalol.

Antiarrhythmic agents, in general, have a narrow therapeutic index. As a result, they are often susceptible to drug interactions with anesthetic agents and can cause significant adverse effects (**Table 4**).

Drug	Action	Dose
Adenosine	AV nodal blockade	6–12 mg
Amiodarone	Class III antiarrhythmic	Bolus 150 mg over 10 min; repeat, if necessary, maintenance of 1 mg/min for 6 hours, then 0.5 mg/min Total dose over 24 h ≤2.4 g
Digoxin	Indirect vagomimetic and slows conduction through AV node	0.5–1.0 mg loading (dose 1: 50%; 25% at 4 hourly intervals; then 0.125–0.25 mg daily) Digoxin levels must be monitored for toxicity (therapeutic blood level: 0.8–2.0 ng/mL; if >3 ng/ml is indicative of toxicity)
Diltiazem	Ca channel antagonist	20 mg × 1 min (0.25 mg/kg) 0.125 mg/kg
Esmolol	Ultrashort-acting β-blocker	150–500 μg/kg × 1 min. 50–200 μg/kg/min
Isoproterenol	β-agonist	2–20 μg/min (0.02–0.15 μg/kg/min)
Lidocaine	Na channel action decreasing duration of action potential	1.0–1.5 mg/kg; 1–4 mg/min (20–50 μg/kg/min)
Propranolol	β-blocker	0.5–3 mg (10–30 μg/kg) q 2 min to max 6–10 mg
verapamil	Ca channel antagonist	5–10 mg. Repeat bolus if needed (maximum dose 30 mg)
Procainamide	Class Ia antiarrhythmic	20–50 mg/min or 100 mg every 5 min until arrhythmia is controlled, QRS prolonged by 50% of original width, hypotension occurs, or total cumulative dose of 17 mg/kg
Sotalol	Class III antiarrhythmic	75 mg over 5 h

Table 3.
The main intravenous agents useful in management of intraoperative arrhythmias.

Antiarrhythmic drugs	Interaction with anesthetic agents
adenosine	• Vasodilation with isoflurane and central neuraxial block • Bronchoconstriction with neostigmine • Asystole with neostigmine, dexmedetomidine, and opioids • Antagonism with aminophylline
digoxin	• Bradycardia is potentiated by halothane and succinylcholine • Caution when using calcium and diuretics (digoxin toxicity)
β blocker	• Myocardial depression with halothane • Bronchoconstriction with neostigmine and atracurium
quinidine	• Prolongs the effects of neuromuscular blocking agents
procainamide	• Antagonizes neostigmine
calcium channel blocker	• Bradycardia and myocardial depression with halogenated agents and dantrolene • Potentiates neuromuscular blockers
lidocaine	• Potentiates the sympathetic blockade of opioids

Table 4.
Antiarrhythmics and its interaction with anesthetics agents.

6.2 Pacing and cardiac electroversion

Both cardiac pacing and electroversion provide a more prompt therapeutic effect and easier dose titration (i.e., pacing mode, rate, current) than with drugs

[8, 18]. They have advantages over drugs for the management of intraoperative arrhythmias.

Pacing is considered in patients with symptomatic bradycardia when a pulse is present but not responded to atropine or second-line drugs (e.g., adrenaline and dopamine) [19]. Temporary cardiac pacing is used in cardiac surgery to increase heart rate, suppress bradycardia dependent tachycardia, overdrive escape rhythms, suppress atrial or ventricular extrasystoles, and terminate re-entrant SVT or atrial flutter. Transcutaneous pacing is used if invasive pacing is not feasible or is impractical.

Cardiac electroversion includes cardioversion (synchronized shocks) or defibrillation (nonsynchronized shocks) of hemodynamically unstable patients, which use high-energy capacitor discharges to simultaneously depolarize all excitable myocardium to terminate arrhythmias. It is highly effective and avoids the potential complications of drug therapy [20]. Defibrillation or unsynchronized cardioversion is indicated in any patients with pulseless ventricular tachycardia or ventricular fibrillation whereas synchronized cardioversion is utilized for the treatment of persistently unstable tachyarrhythmias in patients without loss of pulse. In synchronized cardioversion, the direct current electrical discharge is synchronized with the R or S wave of the QRS complex, avoiding the energy delivery near the apex of T wave, which coincides with a vulnerable period of induction of ventricular fibrillation. The recent use of biphasic cardioversion has shown that less energy is required to convert an arrhythmia to a sinus rhythm. It results in fewer delivered shocks to the patient, less cumulative energy delivered, and less myocardial tissue damage than is found with higher voltage shocks.

6.3 Management of arrhythmias during anesthesia and surgery

Cardiac arrhythmias may not always require treatment. However, the distinction between benign and malignant arrhythmias which carry the risk of sudden death is fundamental [21]. **Figure 2** provides an algorithm for the evaluation and management of rhythm disturbances.

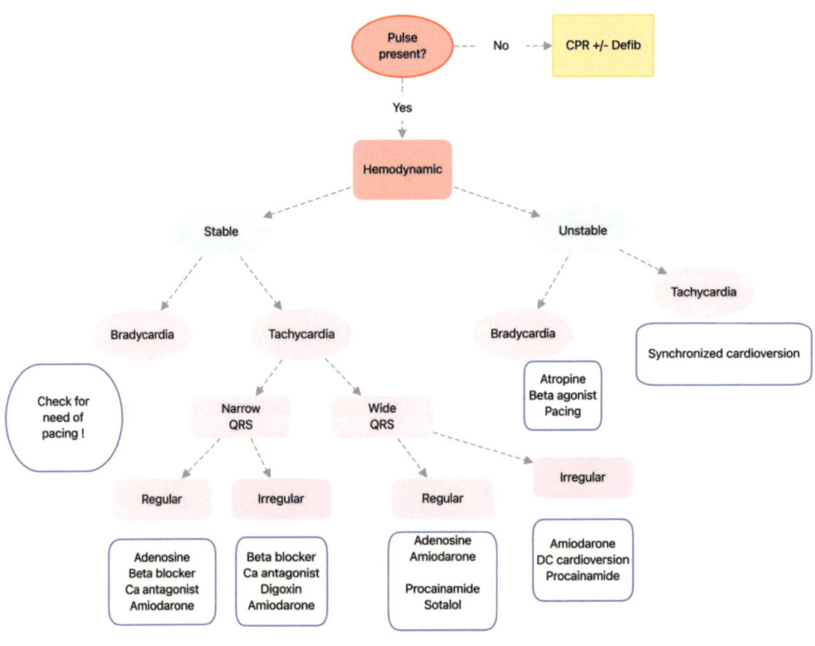

Figure 2.
Management of arrhythmias developed during anesthesia and surgery.

DOI: http://dx.doi.org/10.5772/intechopen.101371

Bradyarrhythmia		**Tachyarrhythmia**		
Sinus arrhythmia	**Conduction defects**	**Sinus arrhythmia**	**Supraventricular arrhythmias**	**Ventricular arrhythmias**
Sinus bradycardia	AV-blocks 1. First degree AV-block 2. Second degree AV-block 3. Third degree AV-block Intraventricular blocks 1. Right bundle branch block (RBBB) or Left bundle branch block (LBBB) 2. Fascicular block. • Left anterior hemi-block (LAHB) • Left posterior hemi-block (LPHB) 3. Bifascicular block 4. Trifascicular block	Sinus tachycardia	1. Premature atrial contraction 2. Paroxysmal supraventricular tachycardia 3. Atrial flutter 4. Atrial fibrillation	1. Premature ventricular contractions (PVCs) 2. Ventricular tachycardia (VT) 3. Ventricular fibrillation 4. Torsade de pointes

Table 5.
Classification of bradyarrhythmia and tachyarrhythmia.

Arrhythmias are broadly classified as bradyarrhythmia and tachyarrhythmia (**Table 5**).

Strategies for clinical care of a patient with bradyarrhythmia (**Figure 3A**) and tachyarrhythmia (**Figure 3B**).

6.4 Bradyarrhythmia

6.4.1 Conduction defects

AV conduction block can occur in the settings of intrinsic cardiac disease, acute myocardial ischemia, general anesthetics, electrolyte abnormalities, and excessive vagal tone. In cardiac surgery, high-grade AV block is not so uncommon complication and thus, a temporary epicardial pacing system is necessary. AV block is classified as first, second, and third-degree (complete). First-degree AV block is generally benign, often needs no treatment apart from careful observation for progression to a higher degree of the block that requires prompt treatment. The second-degree AV block is divided into Mobitz type I and II. In Mobitz type I, the block is often transient and asymptomatic. In Mobitz type II, the block is often symptomatic and has a less favorable prognosis because there is a potential risk of progression to third-degree heart block. Pacing is required if there is severe bradycardia with hemodynamic insufficiency. Third-degree AV block is characterized by electrical instability and may evolve towards asystole. There is no apparent relationship exists between the P waves and QRS complexes. Pacing is typically required because no conduction to ventricles occurs with atrial activity more rapid than ventricular activity (approximately 20–40 beats/min). These bradyarrhythmia (Mobitz type II and third-degree heart block) are not likely to be responsive to atropine and should be treated with transcutaneous pacing or isoproterenol infusion acting as a "chemical pacemaker" while the patient is prepared for transvenous pacing.

Intraventricular conduction defects are generally classified as LBBB, RBBB, or Hemiblock. Intraventricular blocks may be of a His bundle branch block pattern, a fascicular block pattern, or both and result from significant slowing or interruption

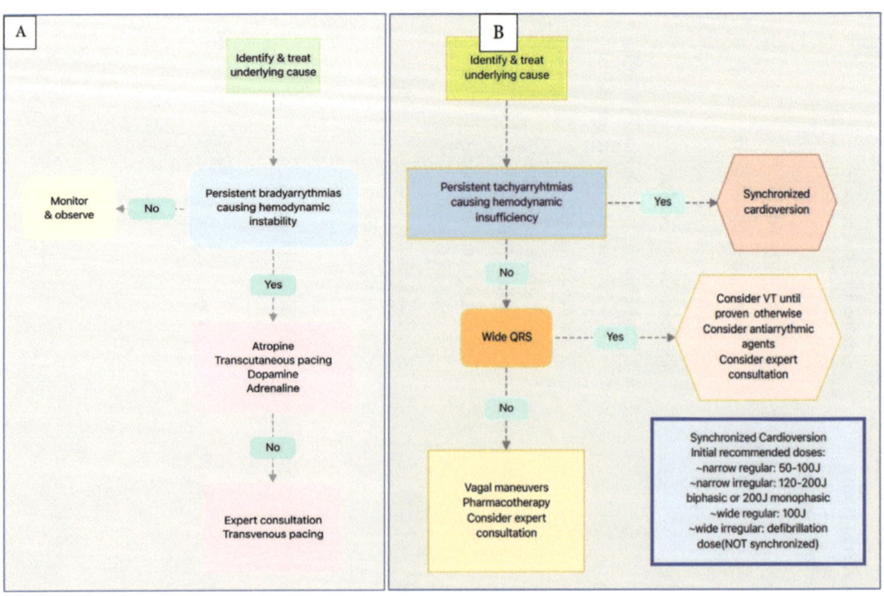

Figure 3.
Algorithm for (A) bradyarrhythmia. Algorithm for (B) tachyarrhythmias. VT: ventricular tachycardia.

of conduction. They are frequently seen in those with and without cardiac disease. In the vast majority of cases, RBBB may be a normal variant with little or no impact on cardiovascular prognosis. LBBB is a more serious conduction disturbance and is always associated with significant heart disease. In the presence of LBBB, acute myocardial infarction is difficult to diagnose. When the LBBB occurs in myocardial infarction, a complete heart block may develop. The anatomical or functional block in a fascicle causes a fascicular block. The left anterior hemiblock is common, while the left posterior hemiblock is uncommon. The combination of RBBB with left anterior or posterior hemiblock is called bifascicular block. Trifascicular block refers to a block of both the left and right bundles or to first- or second-degree AV block with additional bifascicular block. Patients with bifascicular and trifascicular blocks are at risk of a slow progression to an advanced or complete AV block.

6.5 Tachyarrhythmia

Tachyarrhythmias are classified into two categories (narrow complex supraventricular tachycardia and wide complex tachycardia), based on the appearance of QRS complex, heart rate, and regularity.

6.5.1 Supraventricular arrhythmias

6.5.1.1 Premature atrial contractions (PACs)

PACs are a common kind of arrhythmia characterized by early (premature) ectopic beats originating in the atria, which may be seen in patients with heart and chronic lung diseases, sepsis, shock, use of volatile agents, sympathetic stimulation, and excessive alcohol, nicotine, or caffeine. PAC is usually hemodynamically insignificant and self-limiting. But when they are in excess or compromise the cardiovascular function, β-blockers, digitalis or calcium channel blockers can be used after excluding the underlying causes.

6.5.1.2 Paroxysmal supraventricular tachycardia (PSVT)

PSVT is due to the rapid electrical discharge from an ectopic atrial focus, causing regular and consecutive atrial extrasystoles or may be caused by reentry in the AV node by the accessory pathway (AVNRT). It occurs most commonly in normal individuals, who may show no clinical evidence of heart disease. Less common causes of PSVT are rheumatic valvular heart disease, pulmonary embolism, cardiac surgery, thyrotoxicosis, and coronary artery disease. PSVT is characterized by rapid regular atrial rhythm at a rate of 160–220 beats/min, usually with a narrow QRS complex and lacking the P wave. It is typically rapid in onset and conclusion. The majority of patients who develop intraoperative PSVT maintain hemodynamic stability and do not require electrical direct current (DC) cardioversion. For this reason, heart rate control is the mainstay of the therapy that does not require immediate cardioversion [19]. PSVT can be confused with sinus tachycardia, atrial fibrillation, atrial flutter, and ventricular tachycardia. Carotid sinus massage can abruptly terminate the arrhythmia by activation of baroreceptors in the carotid sinus, resulting in increased vagal activity and transient AV nodal conduction block. This aids differentiation between PSVT, atrial flutter, and fibrillation. The Valsalva maneuver can also be used. If these vagal maneuvers are unsuccessful, then rapid intravenous adenosine in a dose of 6–12 mg is the drug of choice for terminating the re-entrant variety of PSVT arrhythmia. Adenosine slows the sinoatrial and AV nodal conduction and prolongs refractoriness, which is very effective in terminating PSVT. Its ultrashort duration of action (10 s) and very rapid onset of action (15–30 s) make it desirable over other intravenous drugs. However, atrial flutter and atrial fibrillation do not respond to adenosine. Other intravenous drugs that are useful for terminating PSVT are verapamil, diltiazem, and β-blockers. Intravenous digoxin is not clinically useful in the acute control of PSVT because of its delayed peak effect and a narrow therapeutic index. DC cardioversion is indicated for PSVT unresponsive to drug therapy or PSVT associated hemodynamic deterioration. Radiofrequency ablation is the preferred approach for patients with persistent symptomatic re-entry PSVT.

6.5.1.3 Atrial flutter

Atrial flutter is due to electrical impulse re-entry into the atria, often giving an atrial rate of 250–350 beats/min with a ventricular rate of 150 beats/min. It is usually associated with varying degrees of AV block, manifesting 2:1–4:1 AV conduction. The rapid P waves create a classic saw tooth appearance on ECG (best seen in leads II, III, aVF, and V_1) and are called flutter waves (F waves). Normal T waves are lost in F waves. Atrial flutter often occurs in association with other arrhythmias such as AF. It usually signifies the presence of underlying severe heart disease and exacerbation of a chronic condition such as pulmonary disease, thyrotoxicosis, or after cardiac surgery. In many instances, treatment of the underlying disease process restores sinus rhythm. Intraoperative management of atrial flutter depends on the hemodynamic stability of the patient. Synchronized cardioversion using a low energy current (50–100 J) is the treatment of choice if the hemodynamic deterioration is present. If vital signs are stable, intravenous amiodarone, diltiazem or verapamil may convert the flutter to normal sinus rhythm.

6.5.1.4 Atrial fibrillation (AF)

AF is much commoner than an atrial flutter, and is one of the most common of all arrhythmias, especially in the elderly population [20, 22]. It accounts for more than 90% of supraventricular arrhythmia in the perioperative setting. AF has an irregularly irregular rhythm. The absence of P waves and variable QRS complexes on ECG is diagnostic of AF. AF is due to excessively rapid and disorganized atrial electrical activation without effective atrial contraction at a higher ventricular rate. The loss of atrial contraction may lead to a decrease in cardiac output and blood pressure that is often hemodynamically clinically significant. Other complications of AF include heart failure, pulmonary and systemic thromboembolism, and a significant risk of cerebrovascular events. Patients with ischemic heart disease, rheumatic heart disease, hypertension, thyrotoxicosis, and pneumonia are more prone to develop AF. The immediate intraoperative management of AF should begin with an assessment of hemodynamic status and correction of precipitating factors. The onset of AF or faster rates of chronic AF during the intraoperative period may be precipitated by acid-base and electrolyte abnormalities, hypovolemia, myocardial ischemia, sepsis, and surgical manipulation in the thoracic cavity. The goal of management is directed towards the control of ventricular response rate with pharmacological agents that slow AV node conduction. IV β-blockers or calcium channel blockers produce rapid control of rate. In the acute setting, the usefulness of digoxin is limited due to slow onset and low efficacy in high adrenergic states such as surgery. Amiodarone is a good choice for rate and rhythm control in patients with AF in the operating room. This agent also suppresses atrial ectopy and thus, recurrent AF and improves the success rate of electrical cardioversion. In cardiovascular compromised patients, synchronized DC cardioversion at 100–200 J (biphasic) is the most reliable method of converting AF to sinus rhythm. However, it should not be used in AF of more than 48-h duration without at least 3 weeks of anticoagulation, attempts to restore sinus rhythm may increase the risk of atrial blood clot formation and systemic thromboembolism.

6.5.2 Ventricular arrhythmias

Ventricular arrhythmias during anesthesia are more common in patients with underlying cardiac disease. Their occurrence must be considered life-threatening.

6.5.2.1 Ventricular extrasystole or premature ventricular contractions (PVCs)

PVCs are commonly seen during anesthesia and can be caused by multiple factors such as electrolyte and acid-base disorders, hypoxia, hypercarbia, hypothermia, anesthetic agents, sympathomimetic drugs, and very commonly direct laryngoscopy and tracheal intubation. They are also frequently observed during cardiac and thoracic surgical procedures. PVCs are ectopic beats arising from below the AV node and give rise to a wide and bizarre QRS complex. PVCs can be unifocal, multifocal, or they can alternate with sinus beats in every second (bigeminy) or every third (trigeminy) beat pattern. The management of PVCs should focus on the correction of underlying problems. Asymptomatic or healthy patients generally do not require any treatment. Frequent PVCs, multifocal PVCs, and PVCs occurring on the T wave should be considered a potentially serious event as they can precede runs of life-threatening ventricular tachycardia or fibrillation and require prompt treatment. The immediate availability of a defibrillator is paramount in the event of a deterioration in the rhythm. Lidocaine is the drug of choice. Amiodarone is also helpful. Propanolol, procainamide, and quinidine are other drugs that can be given to abolish PVCs. However, these anti-arrhythmic drugs (classes I and III) may have proarrhythmic effects, particularly in patients with underlying heart disease [23]. Early and continuous vigilance is necessary throughout therapy. It is important to ensure that serum electrolytes (especially potassium) are kept well within the normal range. Cardiac function should be optimized and cardiac ischemia should be managed aggressively. The drugs should be prescribed only if the overall effect is clearly beneficial. Furthermore, the Cardiac Arrhythmia Suppression Trial (CAST) shows that proarrhythmic death can occur even when PVCs are apparently eliminated. Occasionally, PVCs are induced when there is severe bradycardia. Atropine, isoproterenol, or pacing may be effective to abolish the PVCs by speeding up the SA node.

6.5.2.2 Ventricular tachycardia (VT)

VT is a severe, potentially life-threatening arrhythmia as the rhythm can degenerate into ventricular fibrillation, requiring emergent treatment. The ECG shows a rapid ventricular rhythm with broad abnormal QRS complexes. The ratio of P and QRS has no fixed relationship because of atrioventricular dissociation. Like other forms of arrhythmias, the correction of precipitating factors assumes great importance. It can be categorized into non-sustained and sustained ventricular tachycardia [24].

Non-sustained VT (NSVT) is defined as 3 or more PVCs that occur at a rate of more than 120 beats/min and lasting less than 30s without hemodynamic compromise. These arrhythmias are routinely seen in the absence of cardiac disease and may not require drug therapy. However, NSVT should be monitored carefully, as it can generate into a non-perfusing rhythm.

Sustained VT presents with a broad QRS complex that may be monomorphic or polymorphic. Timely termination of VT is desirable even if it is well-tolerated. Amiodarone is the first-line recommended therapy for patients with VT. The alternative pharmacological therapy includes lidocaine and procainamide. Patients may show signs of inadequate perfusion with or without a pulse. Pulseless VT should be treated immediately with defibrillation and initiation of cardiopulmonary resuscitation according to Advanced Cardiac Life Support (ACLS) algorithm, whereas VT with a pulse should be treated with synchronized cardioversion.

6.5.2.3 Ventricular fibrillation (VF)

This arrhythmia is characterized by very rapid, chaotic, grossly irregular, and disorganized broad complexes on the ECG with no mechanical effect, resulting either from rapid discharges of impulses from one or more ventricular foci or from multiple wandering re-enters circuits in the ventricles. On the ECG, the QRS is absent. It is a serious, life-threatening rhythm due to lack or no cardiac output during the arrhythmia. Clinically, pulses will be impalpable and there will be an acute drop in oxygen saturation on pulse oximetry.

VF during anesthesia and surgery is a critical event. The common causes are myocardial ischemia, hypoxia, hypothermia, metabolic electrolyte imbalance, and drug effects. Management includes prompt initiation of cardiopulmonary resuscitation. External defibrillation is the only effective method to convert VF to a viable rhythm. The most important factor affecting survival in patients experiencing VF is time to defibrillation. Survival is best if defibrillation occurs within 3–5 min of cardiac arrest.

As with any pulseless arrest, contributing factors must be investigated and addressed. When VF is refractory to electrical treatment, IV administration of adrenaline 1 mg or amiodarone 150–300 mg may improve the response to electrical defibrillation. Adjunctive therapy with amiodarone, lidocaine, or magnesium may be indicated. A precordial thump is occasionally effective in the termination of VF but should only be attempted if a defibrillator is not immediately available [25]. Standard ACLS algorithms should be followed for electrical, pharmacological, and adjunct therapy.

6.5.2.4 Torsades de pointes (TdP)

It is an atypical polymorphic form of VT characterized by a constantly changing/twisting QRS axis around the baseline. A non-uniform delay in repolarization is the underlying electrophysiological derangement, manifested as prolonged QT interval on ECG. Tdp is usually short in duration and spontaneously reverts to sinus rhythm. However, rapidly recurring episodes may degenerate into VF and cardiac arrest [26]. The management of Tdp depends on hemodynamic stability and is initially aimed at correction of the precipitating factors and use of intravenous magnesium as cellular membrane stabilizer:

1. Single episode and hemodynamically stable: intravenous magnesium sulfate is the first-line therapy and helps to prevent recurrent arrhythmias.

2. Multiple self-terminating episodes and hemodynamically stable: intravenous magnesium and consider temporary transvenous overdrive atrial pacing and/or intravenous isoproterenol infusion, to reduce the RR interval and repolarization time.

3. Hemodynamic instability: prompt synchronized electrical cardioversion, and intravenous magnesium.

4. Pulseless arrhythmia: Follow VF treatment approach. Intravenous magnesium should be administered. Avoid amiodarone since it has a proarrhythmic effect because of the additional prolongation of the QTc interval but administer intravenous lidocaine instead.

Lidocaine is the preferred antiarrhythmic drug for TdP, though there is a lack of evidence to support its use. Other antiarrhythmic drugs such as amiodarone, procainamide, beta-blockers further prolong the QT interval and therefore worsen the condition. β -blockers will slow down the heart rate, increasing the risk of TdP.

6.5.2.5 Pulseless electrical activity (PEA)

PEA, previously known as electromechanical dissociation, is a life-threatening, non-shockable cardiac rhythm. It occurs when the electrical activity of the heart persists but does not usually follow sufficient ventricular response to produce a sufficient cardiac output to generate a pulse and supply blood to the organs in the body. While the absence of a pulse confirms a clinical diagnosis of cardiac arrest, PEA can only be differentiated from other causes of cardiac arrest by ECG. This means that PEA includes any pulseless waveform except for VF, VT, or asystole. PEA is often caused by a profound cardiovascular insult which weakens the cardiac contraction and is usually exacerbated by worsening acidosis, hypoxia, and increasing vagal tone (**Table 6**). Further compromise of the inotropic state of the cardiac muscle leads to inadequate mechanical activity, despite the presence of electrical activity and ultimately causing degeneration of the rhythm and death of the patient. Overall, the prognosis of PEA patients is poor and still shows a high mortality rate despite optimum CPR.

Prompt and good quality CPR according to ACLS guidelines to maintain cardiac output until the PEA can be corrected is the first step in the management of PEA, while potential underlying causes are identified and addressed [27]. Once a diagnosis is made, specific therapy to treat the cause should be commenced immediately. This process may involve the decompression of pneumothorax, pericardial drain for tamponade, fluids infusion for hypovolemia, correction of body temperature for hypothermia, administration of thrombolytics pulmonary embolism, and early coronary angiography with percutaneous coronary intervention (PCI) in patients with myocardial infarction. Where it is not possible to determine and/or reverse the underlying cause of PEA, the treatment of PEA is similar to that of asystole. The mainstay of drug therapy for PEA arrest is intravenous adrenaline 1 mg every 3–5 min. The routine use of sodium bicarbonate is not recommended, except in special situations (e.g., severe metabolic acidosis or hyperkalemia). Atropine is generally no longer recommended for PEA as it has not been shown to have a therapeutic benefit. Defibrillators cannot be used to correct this rhythm, as the problem lies in the response of the myocardial tissue to electrical impulses. Although PEA

4Hs	4Ts
Hypoxia	Toxicity
Hypovolemia	Tamponade (cardiac)
Hypothermia/hyperthermia	Tension pneumothorax
Hypokalemia/hyperkalemia (electrolyte disorders) and hydrogen ions (acidosis)	Thromboembolism (coronary or pulmonary)

Table 6.
Factors contributing to the etiology of PEA that is widely thought as 4Hs and 4Ts include as following.

and asystole are often considered fatal arrhythmias, PEA has a slightly better outcome than asystole. Previous data by the National Registry of Cardiopulmonary Resuscitation in 2003 revealed that 10% of hospital patients whose initial rhythm is PEA survive with good neurological outcomes [28].

7. Post resuscitation care

Resuscitation of an intraoperative cardiac arrest victim does not end with ROSC and must be tailored to the needs of the individual patient.

Following ROSC after cardiac arrest, many patients suffer from post-cardiac arrest syndrome, which is a high inflammatory state characterized by brain injury, myocardial dysfunction, systemic ischemia and reperfusion injury, and persistent precipitating pathology [29]. The severity of this syndrome varies according to the duration and cause of cardiac arrest. Management of these patients is challenging and requires a structured approach including restoration of adequate hemodynamics and organ perfusion, optimizing ventilation, treatment of electrolyte abnormalities, glycemic control targeted temperature management, and multimodal prognostication to improve outcomes. Specific therapy is determined by the etiology of arrest and initiating treatment to prevent recurrence [30].

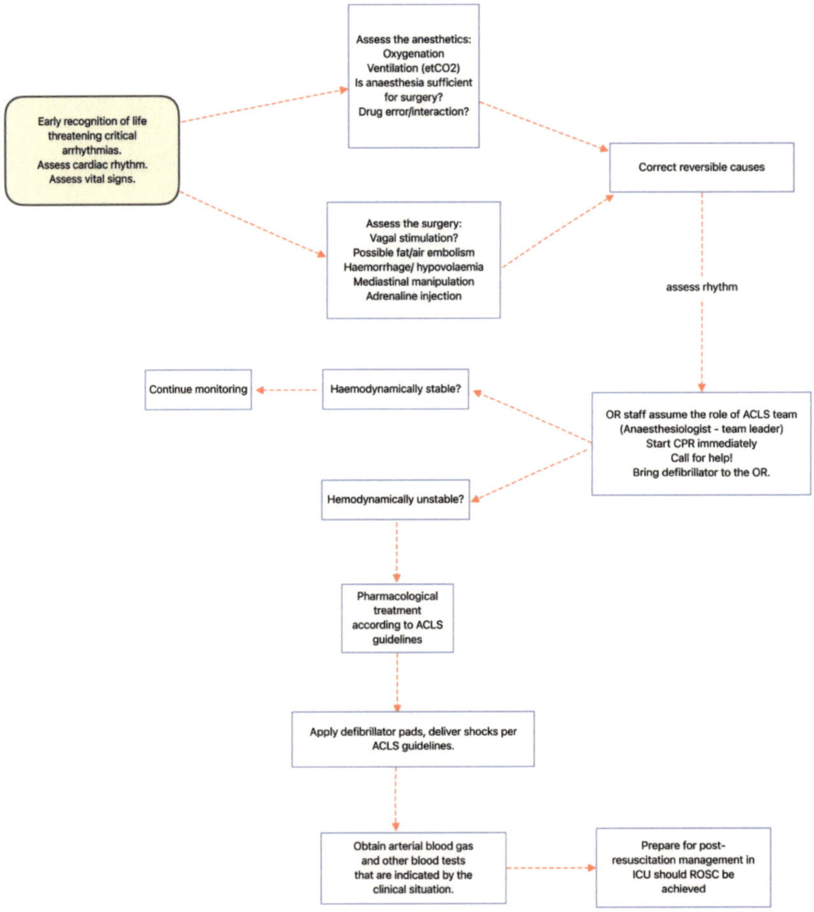

Figure 4.
Summary of management of critical arrhythmias at any time in the operating room [26, 29]. CPR: cardiopulmonary resuscitation; OR: operating room; ROSC: return of spontaneous circulation.

The flow diagram is designed as a step-by-step guide to critical arrhythmias management in the operating room, as shown in **Figure 4** [26, 31].

8. Conclusions

Cardiac arrhythmias can occur in all stages of anesthesia and surgical procedures. They are relatively frequent and continue to be an important source of morbidity and mortality among surgical patients. Most arrhythmias are benign, but some can progress to malignant arrhythmias and necessitate an urgent response. A thorough understanding of the arrhythmias, timely diagnosis as well as performing an early intervention with appropriate therapy enables a proactive approach to patient management and is life-saving for patients.

Conflict of interest

The authors declare no conflict of interest.

Author details

Zuraini Md. Noor
Hospital Serdang, Selangor, Malaysia

*Address all correspondence to: drzuraini@gmail.com

References

[1] Forrest JB, Cahalan MK, Rehder K, Goldsmith CH, Levy WJ, Strunin L, et al. Multicenter study of general anaesthesia II. Results. Anesthesiology. 1990;**72**:262-268

[2] Forrest J, Rehder K, Cahalan M, Goldsmith C. Multicenter study of general anaesthesia III. Predictors of severe perioperative adverse outcomes. Anesthesiology. 1992;**76**:3-15

[3] Katz R, Bigger T. Cardiac arrhythmias during anaesthesia and operation. Anesthesiology. 1970;**33**(2):193-194

[4] Dua N, Kumra VP. Management of perioperative arrhythmias. Indian Journal of Anaesthesia. 2007;**51**(4):310-323

[5] Altinbas A, Tas N, Bektas O. Perioperative arrhythmias. Middle Black Sea Journal of Health Science. 2017;**3**(3):41-48. DOI: 10.19127/mbsjohs.353187

[6] Kennedy A, Finlay D, Guldenring D, Bond R, Moran K, McLaughlin J. The cardiac conduction system: Generation and conduction of cardiac impulse. Critical Care Nursing Clinics of North America. 2016;**28**(3):269-279. DOI: 10.1016/j.cnc.2016.04.001

[7] Methangkool E, Howard-Quijano K, Mahajan A. Cardiac dysrhythmias. Understanding mechanisms, drug treatments, and novel therapies. Advances in Anesthesia. 2018;**36**:181-199. DOI: 10.1016/j.aan.2018.07.008

[8] Toprak V, Yentur A, Sakarya M. Anaesthetic management of severe bradycardia during general anaesthesia using temporary cardiac pacing. British Journal of Anaesthesia. 2002;**89**(4):655-657. DOI: 10.1093/bja/aef240

[9] Feely T. Management of perioperative arrythmias. Journal of Cardiothoracic and Vascular Anesthesia. 1997;**11**(2):10-15

[10] Owczuk R, Wujtewicz MA, Zienciuk-Krajka A, Lasinska-Kowara M, Piankowski A, Wujtewicz M. The influence of anaesthesia on cardiac repolarization. Minerva Anestesiologica. 2012;**78**(4):483-495

[11] Staikou C, Stamelos M, Stavroulakis E. Impact of anaesthetic drugs and adjuvants on ECG markers of torsadogenicity. British Journal of Anaesthesia. 2014;**112**(2):217-230. DOI: 10.1093/bja/aet412

[12] Hunter J, Sharma P, Rathi S. Long QT syndrome. Continuing Education in Anaesthesia, Critical Care and Pain. 2008;**8**(2):67-70. DOI: 10.1093/bjaceaccp/mkn003

[13] Noronha D, Mauricio S, Rodrigues I. Long QT syndrome and anaesthesia. Anaesthesia Tutorial of The Week. 2021;**449**:8 Available from: https://resources.wfsahq.org/atotw/long-qt-syndrome-and-anaesthesia/

[14] Niimi N, Yuki K, Zaleski K. Long QT syndrome and perioperative torsade de pointes: What the anaesthesiologist should know. Journal of Cardiothoracic and Vascular Anaesthesia. 2020;**00**:1-17. DOI: 10.1053/j.jvca.2020.12.011

[15] Fazio G, Vernuccio F, Grutta G, Lo RG. Drugs to be avoided in patients with long QT syndrome: Focus on the anaesthesiologist management. World Journal of Cardiology. 2013;**5**(4):87-93. DOI: 10.4330/wjc.v5.i4.87

[16] Kabade S, Shankar B, Venkatesh Y. Perioperative cardiac arrhythmias: An approach. Journal of Evolution of Medical and Dental Sciences. 2014;**37**(3):9633-9647. DOI: 10.14260/jemds/2014/3247

[17] Kwon CH, Kim S-H. Intraoperative management of critical arrhythmia. Korean Journal of Anaesthesiology. 2017;**70**(2):120-126. DOI: 10.4097/kjae.2017.70.2.120

[18] Part 5:Electrical therapies. Automated external defibrillators, defibrillation, cardioversion and pacing. Circulation American Heart Association. 2005;**112**:IV-35-IV-46. DOI: 10.1161/CIRCULATIONAHA.105.166554

[19] Stewart A, Greaves K, Bromilow J. Supraventricular tacharrhythmias and their management in the perioperative period. Continuing Education in Anaesthesia, Critical Care & Pain. 2015;**15**(2):90-97. DOI: 10.1093/bjaceaccp/mku018

[20] Parida S, Thangaswamy C. Cardiac tachyarrhythmias and anaesthesia: General principles and focus on atrial fibrillation. Indian Journal of Anaesthesia. 2017;**61**:712-720. DOI: 10.4103/ija.IJA_383_17

[21] Part 7:Adult advanced cardiovascular life support. Circulation American Heart Association. 2015;**132**:(suppl. 2):S444-S464. DOI: 10.1161/CIR.0000000000000261

[22] Nathanson MH, Gajraj NM. The peri-operative management of atrial fibrillation. Anaesthesia. 1998;**53**: 665-676

[23] Dan G-A, Martinez-Rubio A, Agewall S, Boriani G, Borggrefe M, Gaita F, et al. Antiarrhythmic drugs-clinical use and clinical decision making: A consensus document from the European Heart Rhythm Association (EHRA) and European Society of Cardiology (ESC) Working Group on Cardiovascular Pharmacology, endorsed by the Heart Rhythm Society (HRS), Asia-Pacific Heart Rhythm Society (APHRS) and International Society of Cardiovascular Pharmacotherapy. European Society of Cardiology (ESC). 2018;**20**:731-732. DOI: 10.1093/europace/eux373

[24] Lorentz MN, Vianna B. Cardiac dysrhythmias and anaesthesia. Revista Brasileira de Anestesiologia. 2011;**61**(6): 798-813

[25] Hines R, Marschall K. Stoelting's. Abnormalities of cardiac conduction and cardiac rhythm. Anaesthesia and Co-existing Disease. 7th ed. Philadelphia, PA: Elsevier; 2018. pp. 151-200

[26] Hutchins D. Perioperative Cardiac Arrhythmias: Part Two. Ventricular Dysrhythmias. Anaesthesia Tutorial of the Week 285. 2013. Available from: https://resources.wfsahq.org/atotw/peri-operative-cardiac-arrhythmias-part-two-ventricular-dysrhythmias-anaesthesia-tutorial-of-the-week-285/

[27] Myerburg R, Halperin H, Egan D, Boineau R, Chugh S, Gillis A, et al. Pulseless electrical activity: Definition, causes, mechanisms, management, and research priorities for the next decade: Report From a National Heart, Lung, and Blood Institute Workshop. Circulation AHA. 2013;**128**(23):2532-2541. DOI: 10.1161/CIRCULATIONAHA.113.004490

[28] Peberdy MA, Kaye W, Ornato J, Larkin G, Nadkarni V, Elizabeth M, et al. Cardiopulmonary resuscitation of adults in the hospital: A report of 14720 cardiac arrests from the National Registry of Cardiopulmonary Resuscitation. Resuscitation Journal. 2003;**58**:297-308

[29] Walker A, Johnson N. Critical care of the post-cardiac arrest patient. Cardiology Clinics. 2018;**36**(3):419-428. DOI: 10.1016/j.ccl.2018.03.009

[30] Ben-Jacob TK, Moitra VK, O'Connor MF. Intraoperative advanced cardiac life support (ACLS) [Uptodate.com]. 2021. Available from:

https://www.uptodate.com/contents/intraoperative-advanced-cardiac-life-support [Accessed: September 18, 2021]

[31] Horvath B. Malignant arrhythmia and cardiac arrest in the operating room. [Internet]. 2021. Available from: https://emedicine.medscape.com/article/2500081-overview [Accessed: August 24, 2021]

Chapter 7

The Initial Assessment and Management of the Post-Cardiac Arrest Patient

Amad Hania

Abstract

Cardiac arrest is the most common cause of death in North America and in the developed world. Advances in care have resulted in improved survival and favorable neurological outcomes in recent times. The initial management and interventions of the post-cardiac arrest patient are reviewed here. Following the return of spontaneous circulation (ROSC) the priorities are to (A) determine and treat the cause of the cardiac arrest, and (B) optimize the cardiorespiratory function of the to prevent further cardiac arrests. The European Resuscitation Council (ERC) and the European Society of Intensive Care Medicine (ESICM) have collaborated to produce post-resuscitation care guidelines for adults following cardiac arrest.

Keywords: resuscitation, return of spontaneous circulation, cardiac arrest, management, targeted temperature management

1. Introduction

Cardiac arrest is the most common cause of death in North America and in the developed world [1]. Advances in care have resulted in improved survival and favorable neurological outcome in recent times [2]. The initial management and interventions of the post-cardiac arrest patient are reviewed here. Following the return of spontaneous circulation (ROSC) the priorities are to (A) determine and treat the cause of the cardiac arrest, and (B) optimize the cardiorespiratory function of the to prevent further cardiac arrests. The European Resuscitation Council (ERC) and the European Society of Intensive Care Medicine (ESICM) have collaborated to produce post-resuscitation care guidelines for adults following cardiac arrest.

2. Determining the cause of the cardiac arrest

In cases of cardiac arrest, the cause determines further interventions that are required. A thorough history and examination can help identify the underlying causes and subsequent interventions required to avoid an imminent threat to life. While cardiovascular disease is a common cause of cardiac arrest, there is a broad range of differential diagnosis for potential causes (**Table 1**).

Cardiac arrest—causes	
• Thrombosis—MI	• Hypovolemia
• Thromboembolism—PE	• Hypoxia
• Tension pneumothorax	• Hydrogen ions—acidosis
• Tamponade—cardiac	• Hyper/hypokalemia
• Trauma	• Hypothermia
• Tablets—drugs/toxins	• Hypo/hyperglycemia

Table 1.
Common causes of cardiac arrest; H's and T's.

3. History

Most patients will not be able to give a history of the events leading up to their cardiac arrest, so it is important to obtain relevant details about the preceding events from any individuals who can give an insight into the patients pre-existing medical condition and the event leading up to the cardiac arrest. These can include family members, friends, witnesses, emergency service personnel, etc. This can help identify the potential cause and help guide management.

4. Physical examination

An initial assessment of the patient is made of the patient using a systematic approach (**Table 2**).

4.1 Airway and breathing

Following the return of spontaneous circulation (ROSC), an initial examination of airway, breathing, circulation, and disability (ABCs) is performed. Airway and ventilation support should continue after the return of spontaneous circulation (ROSC) is achieved [3]. Airway potency is assessed, and endotracheal intubation is required for the patient patients if unable to maintain the airway. If the patient is already intubated, then the position of the endotracheal tube should be checked, as a misplaced endotracheal tube can lead to hypoxia and re-arrest.

Once the patient's airway is secured, an assessment of breathing is to be done. Abnormal examination such as asymmetrical sounds, wheeze, crackles, etc. can help identify potential cause or precipitant. This may reveal potential causes such as pneumothorax, mal-positioned endotracheal, cardiac, and respiratory issues.

4.2 Circulation

Circulation and end-organ perfusion are next assessed. The pulse (weak, thread), blood pressure, skin color (pale, mottled, cold), and prolonged capillary refill time (>2 s) can be indicative of poor peripheral perfusion and the need for IV fluids and vasopressor support. Abnormal cardiac sounds such as the presence of harsh cardiac murmurs, rubs can suggest a cardiac mechanical cause. Diminished heart sounds, jugular venous distension, and hypotension can suggest cardiac tamponade as a potential cause.

a. **Airway**—If the patient is able to speak coherently and is responsive then the airway is patent. Perform either a chin lift or jaw thrust if airway obstruction is identified. A jaw thrust only is preferred if cervical spine injury is suspected, and the cervical spine should be immobilized and maintained in-line.
Foreign bodies, secretions, and facial fractures should be identified if present.
b. **Breathing**—Initial inspection should identify tracheal deviation, an open pneumothorax or significant chest wounds, flail chest, paradoxical chest movement, or asymmetric chest wall excursion. Auscultation of both lungs should be conducted to identify decreased or asymmetric lung sounds.
c. **Circulation**—This is evaluated by assessing the level of responsiveness, obvious hemorrhage, skin color, pulse (presence, quality, and rate), and blood pressure. Capillary refill time can be used to assess the adequacy of tissue perfusion. A capillary refill time of more than 2 s may indicate poor perfusion. Auscultate the heart to identify any abnormalities as described.
d. **Disability**—Assessment of neurological status is made by patient's Glasgow coma scale (GCS), pupil size and reaction, and any abnormal neurological signs. A reduced GCS of ≤ 8 may suggest diminished airway reflexes and may require a definitive airway to help protect the airway.
e. **Environment**—The patient should be exposed to ensure that no injuries are missed.

Table 2.
Initial assessment.

4.3 Disability

A detailed neurological exam is required following the return of circulation to help determine the likely cause and indication for immediate investigations such as a computerized tomography (CT) brain scan. A comprehensive exam may be delayed depending on the use of long-acting sedation and muscle relaxant; however, the presence of asymmetrical neurological findings may suggest intracranial pathology and the need for urgent imaging. Brainstem responses, including the pupillary, corneal, oculocephalic, gag, and cough response to stimulation, correlate with prognostication and survival and should be assessed.

4.4 Environment

An abnormal abdominal examination such as a rigid abdomen, presence of blood in the rectum and stomach can indicative of a surgical emergency and a potential cause. The rest of the patient's body should be examined for the possible source of sepsis, bleeding, and presence of deep vein thrombosis (unilateral leg swelling).

5. Diagnostic tests

Diagnostic tests, including an electrocardiogram (ECG), imaging studies, and laboratory tests, are usually required to help determine the cause of the cardiac arrest, confirm endotracheal tube position, and assess for chest trauma from cardiopulmonary resuscitation (CPR), and to assess the involvement of specific organ systems.

ECG: This can help to identify common causes of cardiac arrest such as acute myocardial infarction (MI), cardiomyopathy, and primary arrhythmia. Following ROSC, a 12-lead electrocardiogram (ECG) should be rapidly obtained and evaluated for signs of ST-elevation myocardial infarction (STEMI) (including a new left bundle branch block) that requires emergency reperfusion therapy. Abnormalities of conduction intervals, the electrical axis may indicate possible etiology, e.g., a prolonged QTc interval may reflect a primary arrhythmia, accidental hypothermia, or an electrolyte abnormality. Evidence of right heart strain (e.g., right axis deviation) may be present in the setting of pulmonary embolus.

In the setting of cardiac arrest, significant coronary artery lesions may be present in the absence of signs of acute STEMI [4]. The incidence of coronary artery lesions is highest in those presenting with arrhythmia such as ventricular fibrillation (VF) or pulseless ventricular tachycardia (VT). Thus, emergency coronary revascularisation may be required for patients without presenting with initial signs of STEMI.

When the diagnosis of the acute coronary syndrome (ACS) is uncertain based on ECG findings, bedside echocardiography may demonstrate focal wall motion abnormalities, suggesting acute or previous myocardial infarction.

Imaging studies: A chest x-ray can identify possible pulmonary pathology and confirm correct positioning of the endotracheal tube and central venous catheter if applicable. Pulmonary edema and evidence of aspiration are common findings after CPR but may be unrelated to the possible cause of the arrest. Pneumothorax may be present as a possible cause of the arrest or may be secondary to the chest compressions, this should be further evaluated and require immediate treatment if indicated. Enlarged aorta or concerning mediastinal findings on chest radiograph may indicate an aortic dissection and should urge prompt CT scan imaging and likely immediate intervention.

FAST examination is the "Focused Assessment with *Sonography* in Trauma" is performed, to identify free fluid in the abdomen and can help to identify possible causes of the arrest that represent ongoing threats to life, including pericardial tamponade, pneumothorax, pulmonary embolism (PE), and intraperitoneal bleeding. Cardiac ultrasound can be used to assess right ventricular size and function (which may be abnormal with PE), determine the diameter of the inferior vena cava (which may be abnormal with a reduced diameter or inadequate dilation following fluid resuscitation can indicate hypovolemia) [5], and assess global cardiac function.

Computerized tomography (CT) of the brain can detect early cerebral edema or intracranial hemorrhage in the comatose post-cardiac arrest patient. This will guide appropriate referral to the neurosurgical unit and may preclude possible anticoagulation administration. A CT of the chest is useful in cases of suspected pulmonary embolism (PE). In cases of traumatic injury, presence of peritonitis, and markedly raised lactate a CT of the abdomen and pelvis can be useful to identify the potential abdominal cause of the arrest.

Laboratory testing: Laboratory can give an insight into the cause of the arrest but also give an indication on the extent of organ damage from the hypoperfusion event resulting from the cardiac arrest. Particularly, electrolyte and acid-base disturbances require close monitoring during the resuscitation and ongoing management following the return of circulation.

Arterial vascular access is frequently obtained in comatose post-cardiac arrest patients given the need for frequent *arterial blood gas* measurements. The frequent use of vasopressor and inotropic drugs for hemodynamic support requires continuous invasive blood pressure monitoring. Arterial blood gasses will give important and immediate data such as acid-base balance, electrolytes disturbance, glucose, and lactate levels.

Serum electrolyte concentrations, including sodium, potassium, chloride, and bicarbonate are monitored as rapid fluctuations in serum electrolytes particularly potassium may occur because of ischemia, acidosis, and catecholamine administration such as adrenaline and noradrenaline through activation of alpha and beta adrenoreceptors [6].

Full blood counts are measured to detect anemia and other hematologic disorders. Profound anemia can suggest blood loss as a factor contributing to cardiac arrest.

Serum troponin is measured to detect myocardial injury. Cardiac arrest, CPR, and defibrillation often cause mild increases in the serum troponin. Rising levels of serum troponin may suggest an acute coronary artery occlusion.

Serum lactate is measured and is usually elevated following cardiac arrest, the rate of clearance of lactate correlates with the likelihood of survival [7]. Lactate should clear over time once reperfusion is restored. Markedly raised serum lactate and rising levels may suggest ongoing intra-abdominal or muscle compartment ischemia.

Specific *toxicology* studies can be of use in patients with a history of drug ingestion, signs of a toxicologic syndrome (e.g., sympathomimetic poisoning), or clinical suspicion of poisoning. For example, myocardial infarction or arrhythmia may be caused by acute cocaine or methamphetamine intoxication. The cardiopulmonary arrest may be precipitated by antidepressant overdose. Sedative overdose e.g., benzodiazepine and opioids may contribute to a prolonged coma independent of any brain injury sustained during the cardiac arrest. The presence of long-acting opioids or benzodiazepine may prompt treatment with the necessary reversal agent for e.g., naloxone for opioids and flumazenil for benzodiazepines.

Hypoperfusion from cardiac arrest can impair kidney and liver function. Frequent monitoring of *liver function tests, and renal function tests* are required to assess organ function which can alter drug prescribing and dosing. *Coagulation tests* are also recommended as blood clotting can become impaired following ischaemic injury to the liver during a cardiac arrest.

6. Respiratory management

Airway and ventilation support should continue after the return of spontaneous circulation (ROSC) is achieved. Patients who are the comatose following return of circulation require endotracheal intubation by experienced operators in airway management. Correct placement of the endotracheal tube should be confirmed by waveform capnography. In the absence of a skilled incubator, it may be reasonable to insert a supraglottic airway device e.g., laryngeal mask, laryngeal tube until endotracheal intubation is achieved [3]. Gastric decompression with a nasogastric tube is indicated to help prevent aspiration.

Patients who have returned normal cerebral function following brief cardiac arrest may not require endotracheal intubation if airway and breathing are normal. Patients should receive oxygen to maintain arterial oxygen saturation above 94% [3].

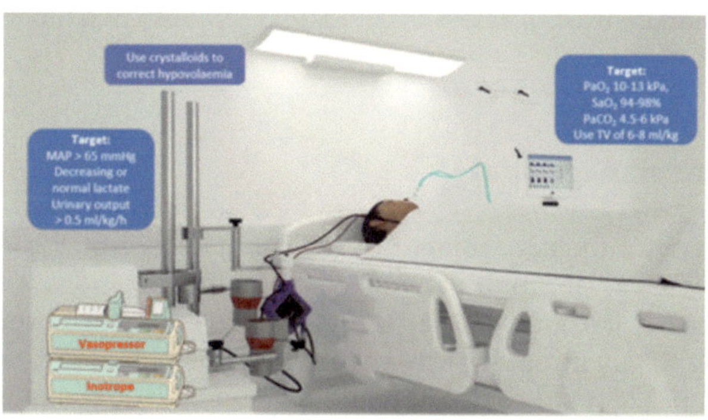

Figure 1.
Haemodynamic, oxygenation, and ventilation targets in patients following ROSC (MAP—mean arterial pressure, PaO_2—partial pressure of oxygen, SaO_2—saturation of oxygen, $PaCO_2$—partial pressure of carbon dioxide, TV—tidal volume).

Patients should receive FiO_2 of 1.0 until arterial oxygen saturations can be measured reliably. Titrate FiO_2 to the lowest level to achieve arterial oxygen saturations above 94% or arterial partial pressure of oxygen (PaO_2) of 10–13 kPa [3].

In patients requiring mechanical ventilation after ROSC, ventilation should be adjusted to target a normal arterial partial pressure of carbon dioxide ($PaCO_2$), i.e., 4.5–6.0 kPa or 35–45 mmHg. This should be achieved using lung-protective strategies e.g. tidal volume of 6–8 mL kg^{-1} ideal body weight, in a unit experienced managing intubated patients on mechanical ventilation (**Figure 1**).

7. Circulation management

Patients should be monitored with an arterial line for continuous invasive blood pressure measurements, and it may be reasonable to monitor cardiac output in hemodynamically unstable patients. Aim for mean arterial pressure greater than 65 mmHg using intravenous fluids, vasopressor, and/or ionotropic support to achieve urine output (> 0.5 mL kg^{-1} h^{-1}) and also target normal or decreasing serum lactate [3]. This may require central venous access.

Emergency cardiac catheterization laboratory evaluation (and immediate percutaneous coronary intervention (PCI) if required) should be performed in adult patients with ROSC after cardiac arrest of suspected cardiac origin with ST-elevation on the ECG or patient's high probability of acute coronary occlusion [3].

Perform early echocardiography in all patients to detect any underlying cardiac pathology and quantify the degree of myocardial dysfunction. Persistent cardiogenic shock not responsive to vasopressors and inotropes may require mechanical circulatory support such as intra-aortic balloon pump, veno-arterial extracorporal membrane oxygenation and for the longer duration a left- or bi-ventricular assist device.

8. Disability management

Patients should be monitored for seizure-like activity using electroencephalography (EEG) to diagnose electrographic seizures in patients with clinical convulsions and to monitor the effects of treatment of seizures. The EEG can also be used in the diagnosis of subclinical seizures in patients under neuromuscular blockade. Treatment of seizures following cardiac arrest should be with levetiracetam or sodium valproate as first-line antiepileptic drugs in addition to sedative drugs [3]. Seizure prophylaxis is not recommended for routine use [3]. Short-acting sedatives and opioids should be used to assess neurological recovery in a timely fashion to allow for prognostication.

9. Temperature management

Targeted temperature management (TTM) reduces neurologic injury and promotes patient survival. Adult patients who remain unresponsive following ROSC from an out-of-hospital cardiac arrest (OHCA) or an in-hospital cardiac arrest (IHCA) with any initial rhythm should have a constant temperature between 32 and 36°C for at least 24 h. Avoid fever (>37.7°C) for at least 72 h after ROSC in patients who remain in a coma [3]. A recent randomized trial (n = 351) investigated TTM at 33°C during 48 h or 24 h in unconscious patients after OHCA [8]. There was no significant difference in neurological outcome between the groups—relative risk (RR) for a cerebral performance category 1–2 at 6 months 1.08, 95% CI 0.93–1.25). Adverse events were more common in the prolonged cooling group (RR 1.06, 95% CI 1.01–1.12). Rewarming should be slow, with a target rate of 0.25°C (0.5°F) every hour (0.25°C/h) until the patient returns to normothermia (37°C [98.6°F]). It will take ≈12–16 h to rewarm. The greatest risks during rewarming are hypotension, hyperkalemia, and hypoglycemia [9]. The complications of TTM include cardiovascular effects such as bradycardia, decreased cardiac output, and vasoconstriction which can lead to a rise in blood pressure [10]. TTM can also cause shivering, increased risk of infection, increased insulin resistance, impaired drug metabolism, decreased gastrointestinal motility, and impaired hemostasis [10]. The routine use of neuromuscular blockade in patients undergoing targeted temperature management (TTM) is not recommended, but may be used in cases of severe shivering during TTM [3]. It is important to be aware of these potential complications of TTM and the known complications need to be recognized for immediate treatment.

10. General critical care management

Provide stress ulcer prophylaxis routinely in cardiac arrest patients may decrease the risk of gastrointestinal bleeding [11]. Provide deep venous thrombosis prophylaxis. Target blood glucose of 7.8–10 mmol L^{-1} (140–180 mg dL^{-1}) using an infusion of insulin if required; avoid hypoglycemia [12]. Start enteral feeding at low rates (trophic feeding) during TTM and increase after rewarming if indicated. Patients should be nursed 30° head-up. This may decrease intracranial pressure (ICP) and decrease the risk of aspiration pneumonia [3].

11. Prognostication

In patients who are comatose after resuscitation from cardiac arrest, neurological prognostication should be performed using a multimodal approach by clinical examination, electrophysiology, and imaging to help inform clinicians and relatives of the likelihood of meaningful neurological recovery.

The clinical neurological examination is central to prognostication. To avoid falsely pessimistic predictions, clinicians should ensure the examination is not carried out with confounding factors such as residual sedation and hypothermia which might give an inaccurate assessment.

The start of the prognostication process begins with accurate clinical assessment ≥72 h from ROSC. In a comatose patient with a motor score of ≤3 at ≥72 h from ROSC, in the absence of confounders, a poor outcome is likely when two or more of the following predictors are present (**Figure 2**) [3]:

- The absence of the pupillary light reflex.
- The absence of corneal reflex.
- The presence of status myoclonus within 72 h.
- Highly malignant EEG at >24 h.
- Diffuse and extensive anoxic injury on brain CT/MRI.

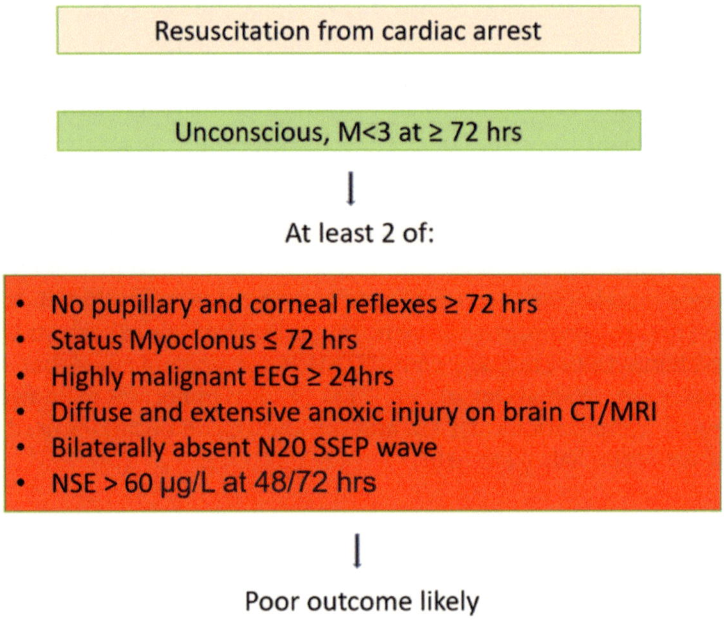

Figure 2.
Summary of prognostication factors resulting in likely poor outcome (EEG—electroencephalogram, SSEP—somatosensory evoked potentials, CT—computerized tomography, MRI—magnetic resonance imaging, N20 wave—negative potential at 20 ms post sensory stimulation, NSE—neuron-specific enolase).

- Bilaterally absent negative potential at 20 ms post sensory stimulation-somatosensory evoked potentials (N20 SSEP) wave.

- Neuron-specific enolase (NSE) > 60 μg L^{-1} at 48 h and/or 72 h.

12. Clinical examination

Clinical examination can be prone to misinterpretation from interference from confounding factors such as sedatives, muscle relaxants, and opioids. The presence of any confounding factors should be excluded to achieve a reliable interpretation from clinical examination of the patient. A motor score of ≤3 in the Glasgow coma score (abnormal flexion or worse in response to pain) at 72 h or later after ROSC, may indicate poor neurological outcome and the need for neurological prognostication. The poor neurological outcome can be predicted by the following test results from clinical examination [3].

13. Neurophysiology

An EEG should be performed on all comatose patients following cardiac arrest. The presence of subclinical seizure activity on EEG in the first 72 h following ROSC is an indicator of poor prognosis. Highly malignant EEG patterns include suppressed background with or without periodic discharges and burst suppression. After cardiac arrest, the EEG is suppressed in many patients but returns to normal voltage activity within the first 24 h in patients who achieve a good outcome [13].

Somatosensory evoked potentials can be performed by electrically stimulating a nerve e.g., the median nerve, and the ascending signals can be recorded from the peripheral plexus brachialis, cervical level, subcortical level, and the sensory cortex (N20-potential). A bilateral absence of the short-latency N20-potentials over the sensory cortex is a reliable sign of a poor prognosis after cardiac arrest with high specificity [3].

14. Biomarkers

Neuron-specific enolase (NSE) is an acidic protease unique to neurons and is sensitive to damage to nerve cells. NSE decreases after 24 h in patients with good outcomes and typically increases in patients with a poor outcome to peak at 48–96 h [14].

15. Imaging

The use of brain imaging studies can help predict patients with poor neurological outcomes. The presence of generalized brain edema, manifested by a marked reduction of the gray matter/white matter ratio on CT brain scan, or extensive diffusion restriction on brain MRI can predict poor neurological outcomes after cardiac arrest. Further signs of diffuse and extensive hypoxic-ischemic brain injury on brain CT include an effacement of cortical sulci and reduced ventricle size [3].

16. Long term outcome in cardiac arrest survivors

Cognitive impairments, emotional problems, and fatigue are common following cardiac arrest [15]. The morbidities can be missed by healthcare professionals. These can have a significant impact on the quality of life of patients and should be addressed for cardiac arrest survivors and monitored on follow-up to allow early detection and intervention with appropriate care [3].

Functional assessments of physical and emotional impairments should be performed before discharge from the hospital to help identify patients requiring early intervention and rehabilitation. Cardiac arrest survivors should be followed up within 3 months post-discharge and be screened for cognitive, emotional problems, and be provided information and support [3].

Author details

Amad Hania
Trinity College Dublin, Ireland

*Address all correspondence to: haniaa@tce.ie

References

[1] Kassebaum NJ, Bertozzi-Villa A, Coggeshall MS, et al. Global, regional, and national levels and causes of maternal mortality during 1990-2013: A systematic analysis for the Global Burden of Disease Study 2013. Lancet. 2014;**384**(9947):980-1004

[2] Benjamin EJ, Virani SS, Callaway CW, et al. Heart disease and stroke statistics-2018 update: A report from the American Heart Association. Circulation. 2018;**137**(12):e67-e492

[3] Nolan JP, Sandroni C, Böttiger BW, et al. European Resuscitation Council and European Society of Intensive Care Medicine guidelines 2021: post-resuscitation care. Journal of Intensive Care Medicine. Apr 2021;**47**(4):369-421. DOI: 10.1007/s00134-021-06368-4. Epub 2021 Mar 25

[4] Reynolds JC, Callaway CW, El Khoudary SR, Moore CG, Alvarez RJ, Rittenberger JC. Coronary angiography predicts improved outcome following cardiac arrest: Propensity-adjusted analysis. Journal of Intensive Care Medicine. 2009;**24**(3):179-186. DOI: 10.1177/0885066609332725

[5] Yanagawa Y, Sakamoto T, Okada Y. Hypovolemic shock evaluated by sonographic measurement of the inferior vena cava during resuscitation in trauma patients. The Journal of Trauma. 2007;**63**(6):1245-1248, discussion 1248. DOI: 10.1097/TA.0b013e318068d72b

[6] Moratinos J, Reverte M. Effects of catecholamines on plasma potassium: The role of alpha- and beta-adrenoceptors. Fundamental & Clinical Pharmacology. 1993;**7**(3-4):143-153. DOI: 10.1111/j.1472-8206.1993.tb00228.x

[7] Donnino MW, Andersen LW, Giberson T, et al. Initial lactate and lactate change in post-cardiac arrest: A multicenter validation study. Critical Care Medicine. 2014;**42**(8):1804-1811. DOI: 10.1097/CCM.0000000000000332

[8] Kirkegaard H, Soreide E, de Haas I, et al. Targeted temperature management for 48 vs 24 h and neurologic outcome after out-of-hospital cardiac arrest: A randomized clinical trial. JAMA. 2017;**318**:341-350

[9] Scirica BM. Therapeutic hypothermia after cardiac arrest. Circulation. 2013;**127**(2):244-250. DOI: 10.1161/CIRCULATIONAHA.111.076851

[10] Leong SH, Chan E, Ho BC, et al. Therapeutic temperature management (TTM): Post-resuscitation care for adult cardiac arrest, with recommendations from the National TTM Workgroup. Singapore Medical Journal. 2017;**58**(7):408-410. DOI: 10.11622/smedj.2017067

[11] Wang Y, Ge L, Ye Z, et al. Efficacy and safety of gastrointestinal bleeding prophylaxis in critically ill patients: An updated systematic review and network meta-analysis of randomized trials. Intensive Care Medicine. 2020;**46**: 1987-2000

[12] American DA. 15. Diabetes care in the hospital: Standards of medical care in diabetes-2019. Diabetes Care. 2019; **42**:S173-S181

[13] Cloostermans MC, van Meulen FB, Eertman CJ, Hom HW, van Putten MJ. Continuous electroencephalography monitoring for early prediction of neurological outcome in postanoxic patients after cardiac arrest: A prospective cohort study. Critical Care Medicine. 2012;**40**:2867-2875

[14] Stammet P, Collignon O, Hassager C, et al. Neuron-specifc enolase as a predictor of death or poor

neurological outcome after out-of-hospital cardiac arrest and targeted temperature management at 33°C and 36°C. Journal of the American College of Cardiology. 2015;**65**: 2104-2114

[15] Orbo M, Aslaksen PM, Larsby K, Schafer C, Tande PM, Anke A. Alterations in cognitive outcome between 3 and 12 months in survivors of out-of-hospital cardiac arrest. Resuscitation. 2016;**105**:92-99

Chapter 8

Prognostication in Post-Cardiac Arrest Patients

Dilok Piyayotai and Sombat Muengtaweepongsa

Abstract

After resuscitation from cardiac arrest, a combination of the complex pathophysiologic process, known as post-cardiac arrest syndrome (PCAS), is attributed to multiple organ damage. Global ischemic cascade occurs in the brain due to generalized ischemia during cardiac arrest and the reperfusion process after the return of spontaneous circulation (ROSC), leading to hypoxic/ ischemic brain injury. Targeted temperature management (TTM) is a well-known neuroprotective therapy for ischemic/hypoxic brain injury. This global brain injury is a significant cause of death in PCAS. The implementation of TTM for PCAS leads to a reduction in mortality and better clinical outcomes among survivors. Prognostication is an essential part of post-resuscitation care. Before the TTM era, physicians relied on the algorithm for prognostication in comatose patients released by the American Academy of Neurology in 2006. However, TTM also announced more significant uncertainty during prognostication. During this TTM era, prognostication should not rely on just a solitary parameter. The trend of prognostication turns into a multimodal strategy integrating physical examination with supplementary methods, consisting of electrophysiology such as somatosensory evoked potential (SSEP) and electroencephalography (EEG), blood biomarkers, particularly serum neuron-specific enolase (NSE), and neuro-radiography including brain imaging with CT/ MRI, to enhance prognostic accuracy.

Keywords: prognosis, cardiac arrest, therapeutic hypothermia, neurological outcomes, hypoxic-ischemic encephalopathy, restore of spontaneous circulation, reperfusion

1. Introduction

Cardiac arrest is the leading cause of ischemic and hypoxic encephalopathy, as the brain is the organ that receives blood from the heart at 25% of all the blood that leaves the heart. Regardless of the underlying cause, patients with cardiac arrest often experience neurological complications, both short-term and long-term. Therefore, neurological monitoring is essential and essential in cardiac arrest patients for proper care and accurate prognosis [1].

The prognostication after cardiac arrest consists of (1) neurological examination, (2) neurophysiologic evaluation, (3) neuro-radiologic evaluation, (4) biochemical markers.

The algorithm for prognostication in post-cardiac arrest (PCAS) patients with restoring spontaneous circulation (ROSC) invented by the American Academy of Neurology in 2006 (as shown in **Figure 1**) has become a landmark guideline [2]. The

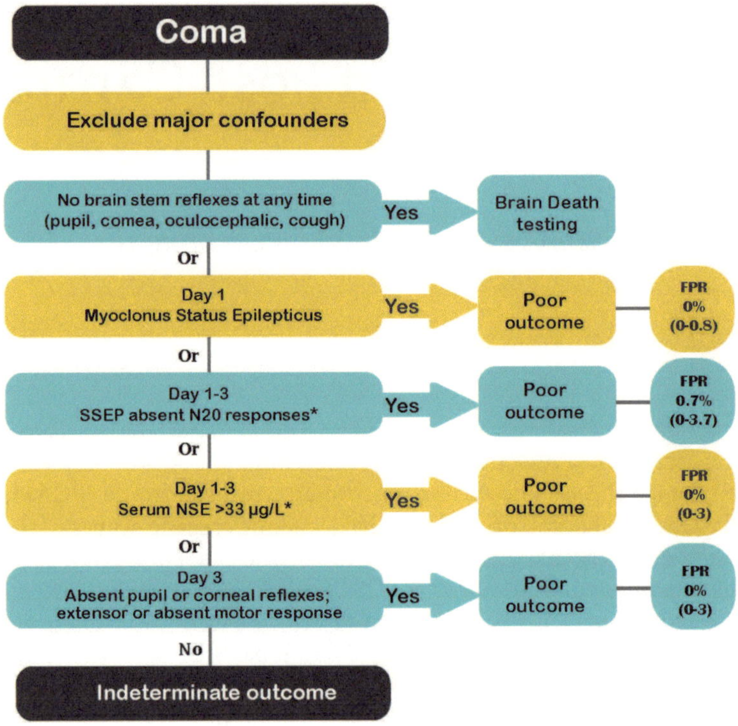

Figure 1.
The algorithm for prognostication in post-cardiac arrest (PCAS) patients with restoring spontaneous circulation (ROSC) was invented by the American Academy of Neurology in 2006.

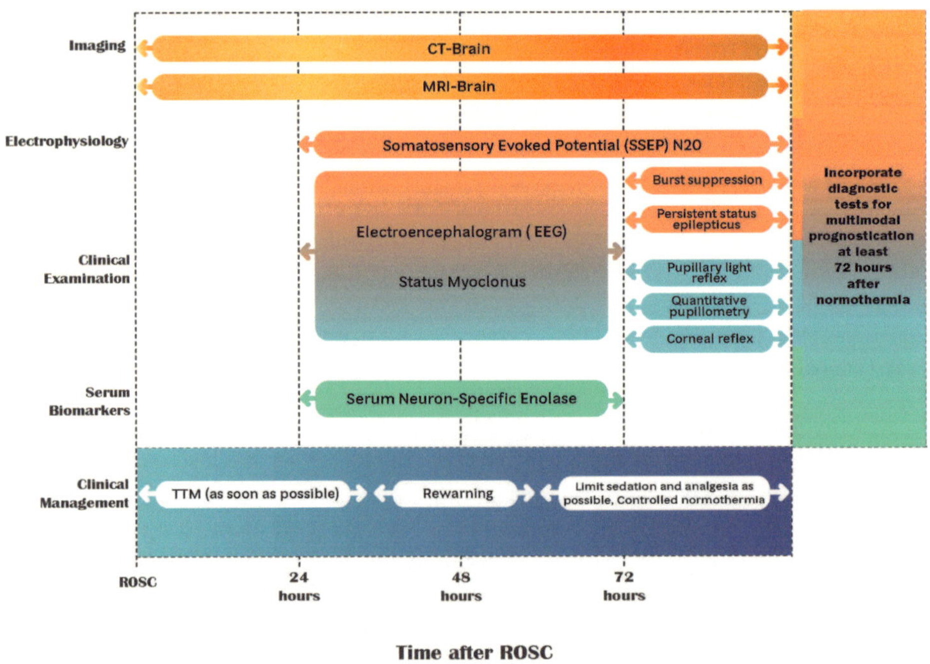

Figure 2.
The algorithm for prognostication in post-cardiac arrest (PCAS) patients with restoring spontaneous circulation (ROSC) was invented by the American Heart Association in 2020.

primary purpose of the algorithm is to determine the poor outcomes for withdrawal of life-sustaining treatment, although most of the PCAS patients fall into indeterminate outcomes. However, due to improved outcomes with targeted temperature management (TTM), clinical and surrogate makers in the algorithm need to be interpreted more carefully in patients treated with TTM [1, 3]. The recent resuscitation guidelines updated the algorithm using multimodal evaluation (as shown in **Figure 2**) to ensure better accuracy in determining the prognosis in post-cardiac arrest patients treated with TTM [4]. The predicting tool for prognostication in post-cardiac arrest patients is available [5]. In contrast, the prognostication in coma patients outside post-cardiac arrest is much less established [6]. In general, for patients who remain coma for more than four weeks, the chance to achieve a meaningful recovery is low.

2. Neurological examination

The neurological examination remains essential for prognostication in PCAS patients, which indicates the degree of hypoxic-ischemic brain injury. Therefore, physicians usually use the overall neurological signs to predict the outcomes after ROSC. The optimal time to predict the outcomes with neurological examination is three days after ROSC in PCAS patients not treated with TTM [2]. In contrast, the neurological examination should get delayed until five days after ROSC or three days after normothermia in PCAS patients treated with TTM [7].

2.1 Glasgow coma scale (GCS)

The initial purpose of the Glasgow Coma Scale (GCS) was to measure the level of consciousness in traumatic brain injuries; however, it is also helpful for predicting outcomes in PCAS [8]. Serial improvement of GCS in PCAS patients is usually associated with good outcomes [9]. Therefore, predicting tools for outcomes in PCAS usually included the GCS [10]. The GCS motor scores less than three at three days after ROSC in PCAS patients not treated with TTM strongly predict poor outcomes (false positive rate 0–3%) [2]. On the other hand, in PCAS patients treated with TTM, the GCS motor scores less than three at three days after normothermia or five days after ROSC may not always predict poor outcomes (false positive rate 19%) [11, 12]. The GCS motor scores more than three before initiation of TTM strongly predict good outcomes [13].

2.2 Pupillary light reflex (PLR)

Intact pupillary light reflex (PLR) indicates proper midbrain function. The absence of PLR three days after ROSC in PCAS patients not treated with TTM strongly predicts poor outcomes (false positive rate 0–3%) [2]. On the other hand, in PCAS patients treated with TTM, the absence of PLR at three days after normothermia or five days after ROSC remains predictive for poor outcomes with a 2.1% false-positive rate [11, 14]. Thus, early absent PLR after ROSC before initiation of TTM may not always predict poor outcomes [15]. Abnormal Neurological Pupil index and PLR quantitative measurements by pupillometry early after ROSC increase accuracy for the predictor of poor outcomes [16, 17].

2.3 Corneal reflex

The corneal reflex indicates the degree of intactness of the pathway from the ophthalmic branch of the fifth cranial nerve through the pons to the seventh cranial nerve and facial muscles [18]. Gently touching the cornea with a thin wisp of sterile cotton will aggravate, leading to involuntary closure of the ipsilateral eye, as well as the closing of the other eye (consensual response). Therefore, the accuracy of the technique is crucial for declaring the corneal reflex present or absent [19]. The absence of bilateral corneal reflex three days after ROSC in PCAS patients not treated with TTM strongly predicts poor outcomes (false positive rate 0–3%) [2]. On the other hand, in PCAS patients treated with TTM, the absence of bilateral corneal reflex at three days after normothermia or five days after ROSC remains predictive for poor outcomes with a 2.2% false-positive rate [11].

2.4 Oculocephalic reflex (Doll's eye movement)

The intact reaction of oculocephalic reflexes (Doll's eye movement) consists of the deviation of both ocular globes towards the opposite direction of cephalic turning. A fully conscious patient does not have oculocephalic reflex due to voluntary suppression. Once an unconscious PCAS patient does not express these symptoms, a lesion must be located at either the afferent or efferent arm of the reflex loop. The afferent arm includes the labyrinthine complex, vestibular nerve (CN VIII), and neck proprioceptors. The efferent arm includes the oculomotor nerve (CN III), trochlear (CN IV), and abducens nerve (CN VI), and their responsible muscles. If the connective pathways between the afferent and efferent arms in the pons and medulla become interrupted in unconscious PCAS patients, the doll's eyes reflex will also be absent. Physicians usually use the lack of oculocephalic reflex together with the absence of other brainstem reflexes to indicate poor outcomes for withdrawal of life support in PCAS patients [20].

2.5 Vestibulo-ocular reflex

Irrigating one tympanic membrane with cold water or saline introduces ipsilateral deviation of both eyes with contralateral fast phase nystagmus lasting for one to two minutes. While switching to hot water produces the opposite reaction: contralateral deviation, with ipsilateral fast phase nystagmus. Bilateral irrigating with cold water or saline gives rise to a downward deviation with upward nystagmus. In contrast, bilateral irrigating with hot water or saline, the opposite reaction occurs. Patients with inflammations and traumatic lesions within the outer and middle ear are contra-indicated to get the vestibulo-ocular reflex test. The absence of any or abnormal responses indicates brainstem dysfunction [21]. The absence of vestibulo-ocular reflex at more than 24 h after ROSC in PCAS patients not treated with TTM usually predicts poor outcomes with a false positive rate of 14% [22].

2.6 Myoclonus status epilepticus (MSE)

Myoclonic movement disorders occurred after hypoxic-ischemic brain injury in PCAS patients entitles post-hypoxic myoclonus. The post-hypoxic myoclonus is divided into the malignant, the so-called Myoclonus Status Epilepticus (MSE), and the benign, the so-called Lance Adam Syndrome (LAS), subtypes. MSE indicates more severe hypoxic-ischemic brain damage than LAS. Clinical features of the post-anoxic myoclonus alone are difficult to discriminate between MSE and LAS. The electrophysiologic studies help enhance the accuracy of the post-anoxic myoclonus diagnosis [23]. The early presence of MSE within 24 h after ROSC in PCAS patients not treated with TTM predicts poor outcomes (false positive rate 0–8.8%) [2]. However, an increasing number of studies report good outcomes in PCAS patients with initial MSE treated with TTM [24, 25]. Therefore, the early presence of post-anoxic myoclonus should not discourage the use of TTM in PCAS patients [25].

3. Neurophysiologic studies

3.1 Somatosensory evoked potentials (SSEPs)

Somatosensory evoked potentials (SSEPs) consist of electronic waves that result from the stimulation of neural structures along the somatosensory tracks. The stimulation sites typically performed for prognostic SSEPs studies are the median nerve at the wrist. The measurement sites are the N20 wave at the contralateral parietal cortex, as shown in **Figure 3** [26]. The artifacts and low amplitude of the N20 wave are the limitations of SSEP interpretation [27]. The absence of N20 wave within three days after ROSC in PCAS patients not treated with TTM strongly predicts poor outcomes (false positive rate 0–3.7%) [2]. An increasing number of cases reported initial absence but the later presence of N20 wave and good outcomes in PCAS patients treated with TTM [28, 29]. Series of SSEPs with the absence of N20 wave until six days after ROSC provide better accuracy for poor outcomes in PCAS patients treated with TTM [30]. Visual Evoked Potentials may be as valuable as SSEPs for outcomes predictor in PCAS patients [31].

3.2 Electroencephalogram (EEG)

EEG has been used together with other prognostic tools for the outcomes predictor in PCAS patients for more than five decades. EEG patterns, which can be found in PCAS patients, include iso-electric, low voltage (less than 20 milli-volts), burst suppression, epileptiform, continuous activity with frequency less than eight Hertz, and continuous activity with frequency less than eight frequency more than or equal to eight Hertz [32]. The first three patterns are considered malignant EEG and predict poor outcomes in PCAS patients [33]. However, malignant EEG alone may not accurately predict poor outcomes (false positive rate **0.9** to **11) (2).** Reactivity

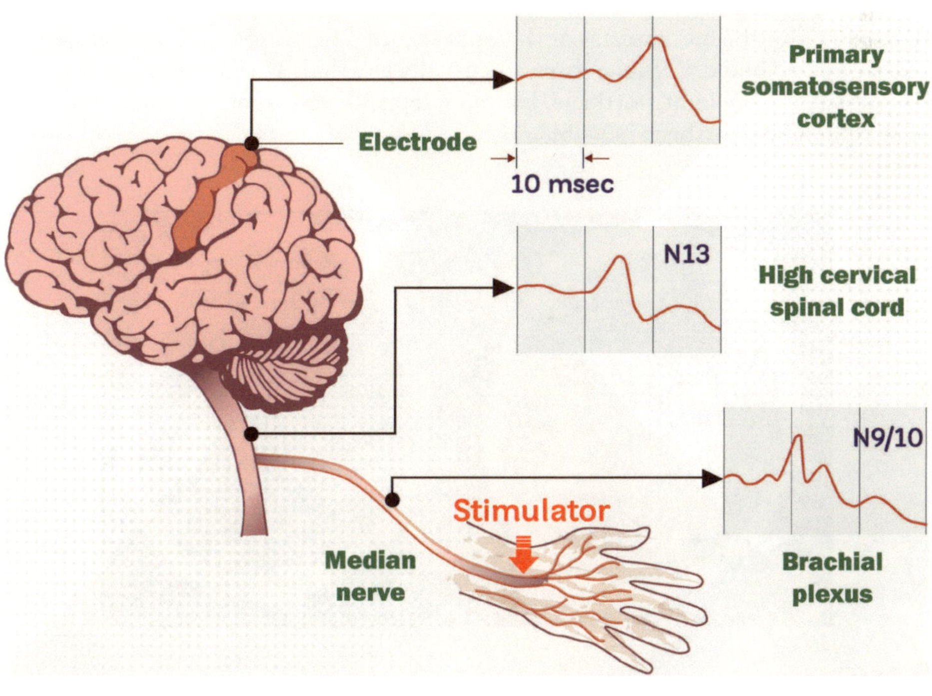

Figure 3.
The somatosensory evoked potential (SSEP).

is a significant change in background EEG activity following external stimuli [34]. EEG reactivity following clapping or sternal rubbing indicates good outcomes in PCAS patients [35].

4. Neuroimaging studies

4.1 Computer tomography (CT-brain)

CT-brain is convenient to obtain early in PCAS patients, and the results are not disturbed by any treatment during resuscitation. CT-brain is beneficial to help determine some neurological causes of cardiac arrests, such as an intracranial hemorrhage. However, CT-brain is not sensitive enough to detect the early phase of hypoxic-ischemic brain injury. The apparent abnormalities such as diffuse cerebral edema with effacement of the basal cisterns and sulci, loss of cortical gray-white differentiation, bilateral hypodensities involving the deep gray nuclei or the arterial border zones (as shown in **Figure 4**), take a few days or weeks to show up in CT-brain [36]. The measurement of gray-white matter ratio (GWR) by the Hounsfield units is helpful to detect the unvisualized early cerebral edema from hypoxic-ischemic brain injury in CT-brain. Many previous studies have shown that if the GWR is low in the CT-brain, it indicates an initial sign of severe hypoxic-ischemic brain injury and a PCAS patient's likelihood of death [37]. The area of the brain used for GWR calculation is varied among studies [38]. In general, the average GWR of less than 1.14 is highly predictive for poor outcomes with 100% specificity and 100% positive predictive value [39].

CT-brain without contrast in PCAS patients with profound brain swelling from severe hypoxic-ischemic insults may mimic subarachnoid hemorrhage [40], as shown in **Figure 5**. Pseudo-subarachnoid hemorrhage was postulated to define this phenomenon [41]. The transposition of edematous brain tissue into the subarachnoid space, transposition of cerebrospinal fluid, and distension of superficial pial veins should be the mechanisms of this appearance CT-brain [42]. Hyperdensity area suspected blood at Sylvian fissure is usually less than 35 Hounsfield unit in pseudo-subarachnoid hemorrhage, but more than 50 Hounsfield unit in actual subarachnoid hemorrhage [43–45].

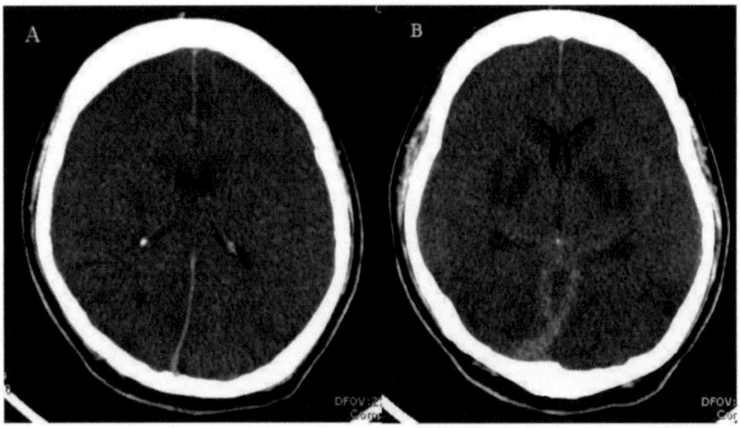

Figure 4.
CT-Brain in a patient with severe hypoxic/ischemic brain injury: diffuse cerebral edema with effacement of the gyri and sulci (A), loss of cortical gray-white differentiation, bilateral hypodensities involving the deep gray nuclei (B).

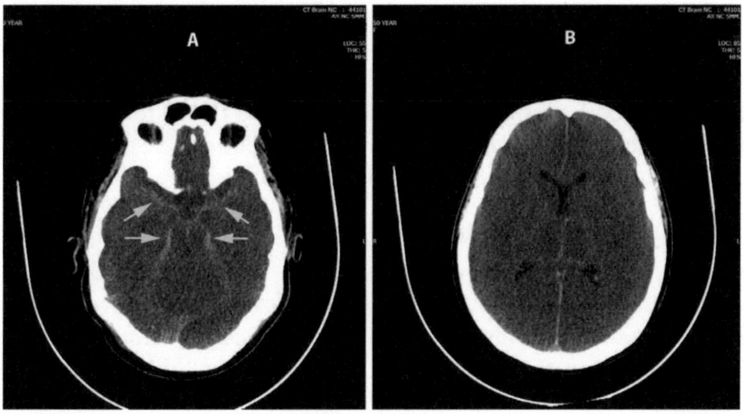

Figure 5.
Pseudo-subarachnoid hemorrhage (A, arrows) in CT-brain without contrast from PCAS patients with profound brain swelling (B) from severe hypoxic-ischemic insults.

4.2 Magnetic resonance imaging (MRI-brain)

MRI-brain is more sensitive than CT-brain for detection of early hypoxic-ischemic brain injury. However, MRI-brain is not as convenient as CT-brain to obtain early in PCAS patients [46]. Diffusion-Weighted Imaging (DWI) sequences of MRI-brain are the most sensitive for cytotoxic injury from hypoxic-ischemic brain insults [47]. Restricted water molecules within ischemic brain tissue cause DWI restriction leading to hypersignal intensity appearance (**Figure 6**) [48]. DWI restriction threshold of 650 x 10^{-6} mm^2/s in more than 9 percent of brain volume determines poor outcomes [49]. Diffusion Tensor Imaging (DTI) plays a significant role in white matter tractography with a similar principle of intercellular water diffusion in DWI [50]. Fractional anisotropy, a DTI parameter, is a quantitative measurement for white matter abnormality [51]. Quantitative whole-brain white matter fractional anisotropy measured by DTI between days seven and 28 after cardiac arrest can predict long-term neurological outcomes [52, 53]. The fluid-attenuated inversion recovery (FLAIR) sequences of MRI-brain can also detect cytotoxic injury from hypoxic-ischemic brain insults [54]. The appearance of hypoxic-ischemic brain injury detected by FLAIR adds up the specificity to DWI in predicting unfavorable outcomes [55].

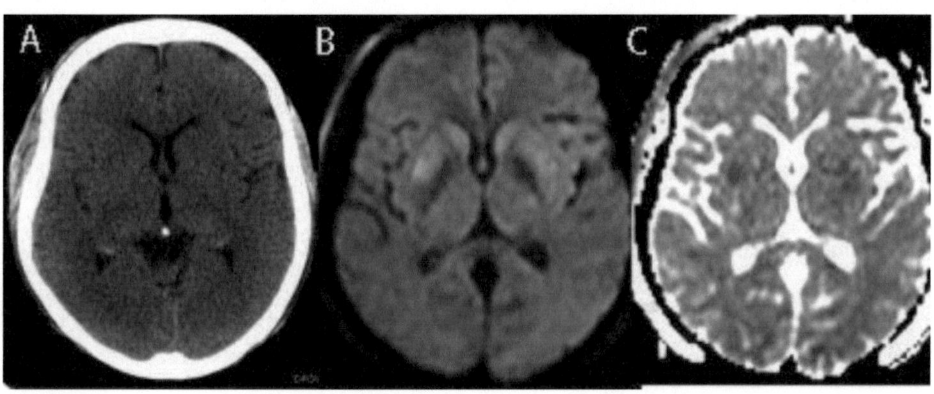

Figure 6.
Imaging of a PCAS patient on five days after ROSC: CT-brain (A) showed no hypodensity lesion, DWI (B) showed hyperintensity in deep nuclei corresponded with hypointensity in Apparent Diffusion Coefficient sequences (C).

5. Biochemical makers

Several previous studies have shown that many chemicals are secreted from the brain into the bloodstream and cerebrospinal fluid (CSF) following hypoxic-ischemic brain insults, including neuron-specific enolase (NSE), S100B protein, Tau, neurofilament light chain, and glial fibrillary acidic protein.

5.1 Neuron-specific enolase (NSE)

NSE is an isoenzyme of the glycolytic pathway found in neurons. Hypoxic–ischemic brain injuries anaerobically upregulate glycolysis, producing and releasing NSE from damaged neurons into the bloodstream [56]. Blood NSE levels were correlated with the severity of hypoxic–ischemic brain injury [57]. Serum NSE is the most useful biochemical marker for cardiac arrest prognostication [2, 4]. In PCAS patients not treated with TTM, serum NSE more than 33 μg/L between 24 and 72 h after ROSC predicts poor outcome (false positive rate 0–3%) [2]. The predictive value for poor outcome (false positive rate 0%) becomes more specific when using the cutoff level at more than 80 μg/L [57]. The cutoff level of serum NSE for poor outcome prediction became inconclusive, ranging from 33 to 120 μg/L in PCAS patients treated with TTM [4]. Serial serum NSE at 24, 48, and 72 h after ROSC was proposed to improve outcome prediction accuracy in PCAS patients treated with TTM [58, 59].

5.2 Other biochemical markers

Other biochemical markers rather than NSE have limited data to use for prognostication in PCAS patients. S100B, a glial-derived protein, more than 0.2 μg/L in serum within 72 h after ROSC may predict poor outcomes [60]. Serial serum S100B at 24, 48, and 72 h after ROSC did not add any predictive accuracy to serial serum NSE [61]. The accuracy of serial serum Tau, a neuron-derived protein, at 24, 48, and 72 h after ROSC is comparable with serial serum NSE for predicting poor outcomes [62]. However, the role of serum Tau fragments, Tau-A and Tau-C, in cardiac arrest prognostication remains uncertain [63]. Serial plasma neurofilament light chain at 24, 48, and 72 h after ROSC with the respective cutoff value of 127, 263, and 344 pg/ml is predictive for poor outcomes [64]. The specificity of serial plasma neurofilament light chain for poor outcome prediction is comparable with other standard methods used in the guidelines [65]. Glial fibrillary acidic protein, another glial-derived protein, is released into the bloodstream only in the presence of pathologic conditions and is more specific to acute brain damage than NSE or S100B [66]. Elevated serum glial fibrillary acidic protein more than 0.8 μg/L at 48 h after ROSC predicts poor outcomes [67].

6. Other tools

6.1 Intracerebral monitoring

Intracranial pressure (ICP) monitoring is rarely applied in PCAS patients. The reliable ICP monitoring techniques, including intraventricular catheter and intracerebral transducer, are solely invasive. Non-invasive techniques using transcranial Doppler, optic nerve sheet diameter ultrasound, and jugular venous pulse pressure are available but have low accuracy [68]. The benefit of ICP monitoring in treatment or prognostication in PCAS patients is uncertain [69]. Persistent elevated ICP above 20 mmHg is usually associated with poor outcomes in PCAS patients [70].

6.2 Autonomic nervous system assessment

Sinus bradycardia during TTM treatment reflects intact autonomic response and predicts good outcomes in PCAS patients [71, 72]. The difference in heart rate during the hypothermic maintenance and normothermic phase of TTM also reflects the intact autonomic response to temperature change and predicts good outcomes [73]. Heart rate variability (HRV) is a conventional method for autonomic function assessment [74]. HRV is feasible to apply in PCAS patients [75]. However, the role of HRV in cardiac arrest prognostication remains uncertain.

6.3 Miscellaneous

The role of aging in PCAS prognostication remains controversial [76]. Advanced age should not be the indication for withdrawal of care in PCAS patients. Also, the role of the pulse index contour cardiac output monitoring system in PCAS prognostication and treatment remains controversial [77].

7. Conclusions

It is essential to determine PCAS patients with poor outcomes for the decision of care withdrawal. There are several methods of prognostication after the cardiac arrest that should be combined to assist in proper prediction. A multimodal approach using Neurological examination, Neurophysiologic evaluation, Neuroradiologic evaluation, and Biochemical markers is recommended to provide the most accuracy for poor outcome prediction. Most of the data used in prognostication studies derive from the out-of-hospital cardiac arrest subgroup. However, the data can be applied to other subgroups of cardiac arrest. Even though a multimodal approach has been used, the prognosis of most PCAS patients still falls into indeterminate outcomes.

Acknowledgements

This work is supported by the center of excellence in stroke from Thammasat University.

Conflict of interest

The authors declare no conflict of interest.

Acronyms and abbreviations

PCAS	post-cardiac arrest syndrome
ROSC	return of spontaneous circulation
OHCA	out-of-hospital cardiac arrest
IHCA	in-hospital cardiac arrest
TTM	targeted temperature management
AAN	American Academy of Neurology
SSEP	somatosensory evoked potential
EEG	electroencephalography

NSE	neuron specific enolase
TCD	transcranial Doppler
GCS	Glasgow Coma Scale
PLR	pupillary light reflex
MSE	myoclonus status epilepticus
LAS	Lance Adam Syndrome
GWR	gray-white matter ratio
DWI	diffusion-weighted imaging
DTI	diffusion tensor imaging
FLAIR	fluid-attenuated inversion recovery
CSF	cerebrospinal fluid
ICP	intracranial pressure.

Author details

Dilok Piyayotai and Sombat Muengtaweepongsa*
Faculty of Medicine, Center of Excellence in Stroke, Thammasat University, Pathum Thani, Thailand

*Address all correspondence to: musombat@staff.tu.ac.th

References

[1] Muengtaweepongsa S. Methods and clinical applications of targeted temperature management. Neurology Asia. 2015;**20**(4):325-333

[2] Wijdicks EFM, Hijdra A, Young GB, Bassetti CL, Wiebe S. Practice parameter: Prediction of outcome in comatose survivors after cardiopulmonary resuscitation (an evidence-based review). Neurology. 2006;**67**(2):203-210. DOI: 10.1212/01.wnl.0000227183.21314.cd

[3] De Georgia M, Raad B. Prognosis of coma after cardiac arrest in the era of hypothermia. Continuum (Minneap Minn). 2012;**18**(3):515-531. DOI: 10.1212/01.CON.0000415425.68900.c6

[4] Panchal AR, Bartos JA, Cabañas JG, Donnino MW, Drennan IR, Hirsch KG, et al. Part 3: Adult basic and advanced life support: 2020 american heart association guidelines for cardiopulmonary resuscitation and emergency cardiovascular care. Circulation. 2020;**142**(16_suppl_2). DOI: 10.1161/cir.0000000000000916

[5] Seewald S, Wnent J, Lefering R, Fischer M, Bohn A, Jantzen T, et al. CaRdiac Arrest Survival Score (CRASS)—A tool to predict good neurological outcome after out-of-hospital cardiac arrest. Resuscitation. 2020;**146**:66-73. Epub 2019/11/16. DOI: 10.1016/j.resuscitation.2019.10.036

[6] Estraneo A, Moretta P, Loreto V, Santoro L, Trojano L. Clinical and neuropsychological long-term outcomes after late recovery of responsiveness: A case series. Archives of Physical Medicine and Rehabilitation. 2014;**95**(4):711-716. DOI: 10.1016/j.apmr.2013.11.004

[7] Matthews E, Magid-Bernstein J, Velazquez A, Falo C, Park S, Claassen J, et al. Prognostic value of the neurological exam in cardiac arrest patients treated with therapeutic hypothermia (S46. 008). Neurology. 2016;**86**(16 Supplement):S46. 008

[8] Mullie A, Verstringe P, Buylaert W, Houbrechts H, Michem N, Delooz H, et al. Predictive value of Glasgow coma score for awakening after out-of-hospital cardiac arrest. Cerebral Resuscitation Study Group of the Belgian Society for Intensive Care. Lancet. 1988;**1**(8578):137-140. Epub 1988/01/23

[9] Schefold JC, Storm C, Krüger A, Ploner CJ, Hasper D. The Glasgow Coma Score is a predictor of good outcome in cardiac arrest patients treated with therapeutic hypothermia. Resuscitation. 2009;**80**(6):658-661. Epub 2009/04/14. DOI: 10.1016/j.resuscitation.2009.03.006

[10] Fugate JE, Rabinstein AA, Claassen DO, White RD, Wijdicks EFM. The FOUR score predicts outcome in patients after cardiac arrest. Neurocritical Care. 2010;**13**(2):205-210. DOI: 10.1007/s12028-010-9407-5

[11] Dragancea I, Horn J, Kuiper M, Friberg H, Ullén S, Wetterslev J, et al. Neurological prognostication after cardiac arrest and targeted temperature management 33°C versus 36°C: Results from a randomised controlled clinical trial. Resuscitation. 2015;**93**:164-170. DOI: 10.1016/j.resuscitation.2015.04.013

[12] Al Thenayan E, Savard M, Sharpe M, Norton L, Young B. Predictors of poor neurologic outcome after induced mild hypothermia following cardiac arrest. Neurology. 2008;**71**(19):1535-1537. Epub 2008/11/05. DOI: 10.1212/01.wnl.0000334205.81148.31

[13] Hifumi T, Kuroda Y, Kawakita K, Sawano H, Tahara Y, Hase M, et al.

Effect of admission glasgow coma scale motor score on neurological outcome in out-of-hospital cardiac arrest patients receiving therapeutic hypothermia. Circulation Journal. 2015;**79**(10):2201-2208. DOI: 10.1253/circj.cj-15-0308

[14] Martinell L, Nielsen N, Herlitz J, Karlsson T, Horn J, Wise MP, et al. Early predictors of poor outcome after out-of-hospital cardiac arrest. Critical Care. 2017;**21**(1):96. DOI: 10.1186/s13054-017-1677-2

[15] Dhakal LP, Sen A, Stanko CM, Rawal B, Heckman MG, Hoyne JB, et al. Early absent pupillary light reflexes after cardiac arrest in patients treated with therapeutic hypothermia. Therapeutic Hypothermia and Temperature Management. 2016;**6**(3):116-121. DOI: 10.1089/ther.2015.0035

[16] Riker RR, Sawyer ME, Fischman VG, May T, Lord C, Eldridge A, et al. Neurological pupil index and pupillary light reflex by pupillometry predict outcome early after cardiac arrest. Neurocritical Care. 2020;**32**(1):152-161. Epub 2019/05/10. DOI: 10.1007/s12028-019-00717-4

[17] Tamura T, Namiki J, Sugawara Y, Sekine K, Yo K, Kanaya T, et al. Early outcome prediction with quantitative pupillary response parameters after out-of-hospital cardiac arrest: A multicenter prospective observational study. PLoS One. 2020;**15**(3):e0228224. Epub 2020/03/20. DOI: 10.1371/journal.pone.0228224

[18] Greer DG, Donofrio PD. CHAPTER 16 - Electrophysiological evaluations. In: Dobbs MR, editor. Clinical Neurotoxicology. Philadelphia: W.B. Saunders; 2009. pp. 201-212

[19] Geocadin RG, Callaway CW, Fink EL, Golan E, Greer DM, Ko NU, et al. Standards for studies of neurological prognostication in comatose survivors of cardiac arrest: A Scientific Statement From the American Heart Association. Circulation. 2019;**140**(9):e517-e42. DOI: 10.1161/cir.0000000000000702

[20] Geocadin RG, Buitrago MM, Torbey MT, Chandra-Strobos N, Williams MA, Kaplan PW. Neurologic prognosis and withdrawal of life support after resuscitation from cardiac arrest. Neurology. 2006;**67**(1):105-108. DOI: 10.1212/01.wnl.0000223335.86166.b4

[21] Rzewnicki I, Łebkowski W, Kordecki JK. Evaluation of vestibulo-ocular reflex in patients with damage to the central nervous system (GCS score 5-3). Advances in Medical Sciences. 2015;**60**(1):107-111. DOI: 10.1016/j.advms.2014.12.001

[22] Peberdy MA, Callaway CW, Neumar RW, Geocadin RG, Zimmerman JL, Donnino M, et al. Part 9: Post-cardiac arrest care: 2010 American Heart Association Guidelines for Cardiopulmonary Resuscitation and Emergency Cardiovascular Care. Circulation. 2010;**122**(18 Suppl 3): S768-S786. Epub 2010/10/22. DOI: 10.1161/CIRCULATIONAHA.110.971002

[23] Freund B, Kaplan PW. Post-hypoxic myoclonus: Differentiating benign and malignant etiologies in diagnosis and prognosis. Clinical Neurophysiology Practice. 2017;**2**:98-102. DOI: 10.1016/j.cnp.2017.03.003

[24] Lucas JM, Cocchi MN, Salciccioli J, Stanbridge JA, Geocadin RG, Herman ST, et al. Neurologic recovery after therapeutic hypothermia in patients with post-cardiac arrest myoclonus. Resuscitation. 2012;**83**(2):265-269. DOI: 10.1016/j.resuscitation.2011.09.017

[25] Seder DB, Sunde K, Rubertsson S, Mooney M, Stammet P, Riker RR, et al.

Neurologic outcomes and postresuscitation care of patients with myoclonus following cardiac arrest. Critical Care Medicine. 2015;**43**(5):965-972. Epub 2015/02/06. DOI: 10.1097/ccm.0000000000000880. PubMed PMID: 25654176

[26] Muengtaweepongsa S. General Principles of Somatosensory Evoked Potentials. 2019. eMedicine, Medscape. 26 Feb 2019. Available from: https://emedicine.medscape.com/article/1139906-overview.

[27] Pfeifer R, Weitzel S, Günther A, Berrouschot J, Fischer M, Isenmann S, et al. Investigation of the inter-observer variability effect on the prognostic value of somatosensory evoked potentials of the median nerve (SSEP) in cardiac arrest survivors using an SSEP classification. Resuscitation. 2013; **84**(10):1375-1381. DOI: 10.1016/j.resuscitation.2013.05.016

[28] Amorim E, Ghassemi MM, Lee JW, Greer DM, Kaplan PW, Cole AJ, et al. Estimating the false positive rate of absent somatosensory evoked potentials in cardiac arrest prognostication. Critical Care Medicine. 2018;**46**(12): e1213-e1e21. Epub 2018/09/25. DOI: 10.1097/ccm.0000000000003436

[29] Habeych ME, Moshayedi P, Rittenberger JC, Gunn SR. Initial absence of N20 waveforms from median nerve somatosensory evoked potentials in a patient with cardiac arrest and good outcomes. Clinical and Experimental Emergency Medicine. 2019;**6**:177-182. Epub 2019/02/12. DOI: 10.15441/ceem.18.015

[30] Sandroni C, D'Arrigo S, Cacciola S, Hoedemaekers CWE, Kamps MJA, Oddo M, et al. Prediction of poor neurological outcome in comatose survivors of cardiac arrest: A systematic review. Intensive Care Medicine. 2020;**46**(10):1803-1851. DOI: 10.1007/s00134-020-06198-w

[31] Choi SP, Park KN, Wee JH, Park JH, Youn CS, Kim HJ, et al. Can somatosensory and visual evoked potentials predict neurological outcome during targeted temperature management in post cardiac arrest patients? Resuscitation. 2017;**119**:70-75. Epub 2017/06/27. DOI: 10.1016/j.resuscitation.2017.06.022

[32] Hofmeijer J, Van Putten MJAM. EEG in postanoxic coma: Prognostic and diagnostic value. Clinical Neurophysiology. 2016;**127**(4):2047-2055. DOI: 10.1016/j.clinph.2016.02.002

[33] Westhall E, Rossetti AO, Van Rootselaar A-F, Wesenberg Kjaer T, Horn J, Ullén S, et al. Standardized EEG interpretation accurately predicts prognosis after cardiac arrest. Neurology. 2016;**86**(16):1482-1490. DOI: 10.1212/wnl.0000000000002462

[34] Liu G, Su Y, Liu Y, Jiang M, Zhang Y, Zhang Y, et al. Predicting outcome in comatose patients: The role of EEG reactivity to quantifiable electrical stimuli. Evidence-based Complementary and Alternative Medicine. 2016;**2016**:1-7. DOI: 10.1155/2016/8273716

[35] Admiraal MM, Horn J, Hofmeijer J, Hoedemaekers CWE, van Kaam CR, Keijzer HM, et al. EEG reactivity testing for prediction of good outcome in patients after cardiac arrest. Neurology. 2020;**95**(6):e653-ee61. DOI: 10.1212/wnl.0000000000009991

[36] Kjos BO, Brant-Zawadzki M, Young RG. Early CT findings of global central nervous system hypoperfusion. AJR American Journal of Roentgenology. 1983;**141**(6):1227-1232. Epub 1983/12/01

[37] Torbey MT, Selim M, Knorr J, Bigelow C, Recht L. Quantitative analysis of the loss of distinction between gray and white matter in comatose patients after cardiac arrest.

Stroke. 2000;**31**(9):2163-2167. Epub 2000/09/08

[38] Torbey MT, Geocadin R, Bhardwaj A. Brain arrest neurological outcome scale (BrANOS): Predicting mortality and severe disability following cardiac arrest. Resuscitation. 2004;**63**(1):55-63. Epub 2004/09/29. DOI: 10.1016/j.resuscitation.2004.03.021

[39] Kim S, Choi S, Park K, Youn C, Oh S, Choi S. Early brain computed tomography findings are associated with outcome in patients treated with therapeutic hypothermia after out-of-hospital cardiac arrest. Scandinavian Journal of Trauma, Resuscitation and Emergency Medicine. 2013;**21**(1):57. DOI: 10.1186/1757-7241-21-57

[40] Given CA, Burdette JH, Elster AD, Williams DW. Pseudo-subarachnoid hemorrhage: A potential imaging pitfall associated with diffuse cerebral edema. American Journal of Neuroradiology. 2003;**24**(2):254-256

[41] You JS, Park S, Park YS, Chung SP. Pseudo-subarachnoid hemorrhage. The American Journal of Emergency Medicine. 2008;**26**(4):521 e1-521 e2. DOI: 10.1016/j.ajem.2007.08.031

[42] Platt A, Collins J, Ramos E, Goldenberg FD. Pseudosubarachnoid hemorrhage: A systematic review of causes, diagnostic modalities, and outcomes in patients who present with pseudosubarachnoid hemorrhage. Surgical Neurology International. 2021;**12**:29. Epub 2021/02/19. DOI: 10.25259/sni_905_2020

[43] Yuzawa H, Higano S, Mugikura S, Umetsu A, Murata T, Nakagawa A, et al. Pseudo-subarachnoid hemorrhage found in patients with postresuscitation encephalopathy: Characteristics of CT findings and clinical importance. American Journal of Neuroradiology. 2008;**29**(8):1544-1549. DOI: 10.3174/ajnr.a1167

[44] Ahn J, Choi S, Jung Y, Min Y. Clinical characteristics of patients with pseudo-subarachnoid haemorrhage who were successfully resuscitated from out-of-hospital cardiopulmonary arrest. Hong Kong Journal of Emergency Medicine. 2012;**19**(2):85-91. DOI: 10.1177/102490791201900202

[45] Choi KS, Won YD, Yi HJ, Lim TH, Lee YJ, Chun HJ. Therapeutic and prognostic implications of subarachnoid hemorrhage in patients who suffered cardiopulmonary arrest and underwent cardiopulmonary resuscitation during an emergency room stay. Clinical Neurology and Neurosurgery. 2013;**115**(10):2088-2093. Epub 2013/08/13. DOI: 10.1016/j.clineuro.2013.07.024

[46] Zhou SE, Maciel CB, Ormseth CH, Beekman R, Gilmore EJ, Greer DM. Distinct predictive values of current neuroprognostic guidelines in post-cardiac arrest patients. Resuscitation. 2019;**139**:343-350. DOI: 10.1016/j.resuscitation.2019.03.035

[47] Obenaus A, Badaut J. Chapter 3 - Noninvasive Imaging Techniques for Brain Edema: From Basic Science to the Clinic. In: Badaut J, Plesnila N, editors. Brain Edema. San Diego: Academic Press; 2017. pp. 51-69

[48] Patil S, Melkundi SS, Govinda RBT. Evaluation of intracranial lesions by diffusion weighted imaging. Journal of Evolution of Medical and Dental Sciences. 2015;**4**:12505

[49] Hirsch KG, Mlynash M, Eyngorn I, Pirsaheli R, Okada A, Komshian S, et al. Multi-center study of diffusion-weighted imaging in coma after cardiac arrest. Neurocritical Care. 2016;**24**(1):82-89. Epub 2015/07/15. DOI: 10.1007/s12028-015-0179-9

[50] Alexander AL, Lee JE, Lazar M, Field AS. Diffusion tensor imaging of the brain. Neurotherapeutics.

2007;**4**(3):316-329. DOI: 10.1016/j.nurt.2007.05.011

[51] Van Der Eerden AW, Khalilzadeh O, Perlbarg V, Dinkel J, Sanchez P, Vos PE, et al. White matter changes in comatose survivors of anoxic ischemic encephalopathy and traumatic brain injury: Comparative diffusion-tensor imaging study. Radiology. 2014;**270**(2):506-516. DOI: 10.1148/radiol.13122720

[52] Luyt CE, Galanaud D, Perlbarg V, Vanhaudenhuyse A, Stevens RD, Gupta R, et al. Diffusion tensor imaging to predict long-term outcome after cardiac arrest: A bicentric pilot study. Anesthesiology. 2012;**117**(6):1311-1321. Epub 2012/11/09. DOI: 10.1097/ALN.0b013e318275148c

[53] Velly L, Perlbarg V, Boulier T, Adam N, Delphine S, Luyt CE, et al. Use of brain diffusion tensor imaging for the prediction of long-term neurological outcomes in patients after cardiac arrest: A multicentre, international, prospective, observational, cohort study. Lancet Neurology. 2018;**17**(4):317-326. Epub 2018/03/04. DOI: 10.1016/S1474-4422(18)30027-9

[54] Saranathan M, Worters PW, Rettmann DW, Winegar B, Becker J. Physics for clinicians: Fluid-attenuated inversion recovery (FLAIR) and double inversion recovery (DIR) Imaging. Journal of Magnetic Resonance Imaging. 2017;**46**(6):1590-1600. DOI: 10.1002/jmri.25737

[55] Lopez Soto C, Dragoi L, Heyn CC, Kramer A, Pinto R, Adhikari NKJ, et al. Imaging for neuroprognostication after cardiac arrest: Systematic review and meta-analysis. Neurocritical Care. 2020;**32**(1):206-216. DOI: 10.1007/s12028-019-00842-0

[56] Haque A, Polcyn R, Matzelle D, Banik NL. New insights into the role of neuron-specific enolase in neuro-inflammation, neurodegeneration, and neuroprotection. Brain Sciences. 2018;**8**(2):33. DOI: 10.3390/brainsci8020033

[57] Almaraz AC, Bobrow BJ, Wingerchuk DM, Wellik KE, Demaerschalk BM. Serum neuron specific enolase to predict neurological outcome after cardiopulmonary resuscitation: A critically appraised topic. The Neurologist. 2009;**15**(1):44-48. DOI: 10.1097/NRL.0b013e318191f810

[58] Stammet P, Collignon O, Hassager C, Wise MP, Hovdenes J, Aneman A, et al. Neuron-specific enolase as a predictor of death or poor neurological outcome after out-of-hospital cardiac arrest and targeted temperature management at 33 degrees C and 36 degrees C. Journal of the American College of Cardiology. 2015;**65**(19):2104-2114. Epub 2015/05/16. DOI: 10.1016/j.jacc.2015.03.538

[59] Ryoo SM, Kim YJ, Sohn CH, Ahn S, Seo DW, Kim WY. Prognostic abilities of serial neuron-specific enolase and lactate and their combination in cardiac arrest survivors during targeted temperature management. Journal of Clinical Medicine. 2020;**9**(1):159. Epub 2020/01/16. DOI: 10.3390/jcm9010159

[60] Jang JH, Park WB, Lim YS, Choi JY, Cho JS, Woo JH, et al. Combination of S100B and procalcitonin improves prognostic performance compared to either alone in patients with cardiac arrest: A prospective observational study. Medicine (Baltimore). 2019;**98**(6):e14496. Epub 2019/02/09. DOI: 10.1097/MD.0000000000014496

[61] Stammet P, Dankiewicz J, Nielsen N, Fays F, Collignon O, Hassager C, et al. Protein S100 as outcome predictor after out-of-hospital cardiac arrest and targeted temperature management at

33 °C and 36 °C. Critical Care. 2017;**21**(1): 153. DOI: 10.1186/s13054-017-1729-7

[62] Mattsson N, Zetterberg H, Nielsen N, Blennow K, Dankiewicz J, Friberg H, et al. Serum tau and neurological outcome in cardiac arrest. Annals of Neurology. 2017;**82**(5):665-675. Epub 2017/10/06. DOI: 10.1002/ana.25067

[63] Grand J, Kjaergaard J, Nielsen N, Friberg H, Cronberg T, Bro-Jeppesen J, et al. Serum tau fragments as predictors of death or poor neurological outcome after out-of-hospital cardiac arrest. Biomarkers. 2019;**24**(6):584-591. DOI: 10.1080/1354750x.2019.1609580

[64] Wihersaari L, Ashton NJ, Reinikainen M, Jakkula P, Pettila V, Hastbacka J, et al. Neurofilament light as an outcome predictor after cardiac arrest: A post hoc analysis of the COMACARE trial. Intensive Care Medicine. 2021;**47**(1):39-48. Epub 2020/08/28. DOI: 10.1007/s00134-020-06218-9

[65] Moseby-Knappe M, Mattsson N, Nielsen N, Zetterberg H, Blennow K, Dankiewicz J, et al. Serum neurofilament light chain for prognosis of outcome after cardiac arrest. JAMA Neurology. 2019;**76**(1):64-71. Epub 2018/11/02. DOI: 10.1001/jamaneurol.2018.3223

[66] Hol EM, Pekny M. Glial fibrillary acidic protein (GFAP) and the astrocyte intermediate filament system in diseases of the central nervous system. Current Opinion in Cell Biology. 2015;**32**: 121-130. Epub 2015/03/03. DOI: 10.1016/j.ceb.2015.02.004

[67] Helwig K, Seeger F, Holschermann H, Lischke V, Gerriets T, Niessner M, et al. Elevated serum glial fibrillary acidic protein (GFAP) is associated with poor functional outcome after cardiopulmonary resuscitation. Neurocritical Care. 2017;**27**(1):68-74. Epub 2017/01/06. DOI: 10.1007/s12028-016-0371-6

[68] Cardim D, Griesdale DE, Ainslie PN, Robba C, Calviello L, Czosnyka M, et al. A comparison of non-invasive versus invasive measures of intracranial pressure in hypoxic ischaemic brain injury after cardiac arrest. Resuscitation. 2019;**137**:221-228. DOI: 10.1016/j.resuscitation.2019.01.002

[69] Sekhon MS, Griesdale DE, Ainslie PN, Gooderham P, Foster D, Czosnyka M, et al. Intracranial pressure and compliance in hypoxic ischemic brain injury patients after cardiac arrest. Resuscitation. 2019;**141**:96-103. DOI: 10.1016/j.resuscitation.2019.05.036

[70] Reis C, Akyol O, Araujo C, Huang L, Enkhjargal B, Malaguit J, et al. Pathophysiology and the monitoring methods for cardiac arrest associated brain injury. International Journal of Molecular Sciences. 2017;**18**(1):129. DOI: 10.3390/ijms18010129

[71] Thomsen JH, Hassager C, Bro-Jeppesen J, Soholm H, Nielsen N, Wanscher M, et al. Sinus bradycardia during hypothermia in comatose survivors of out-of-hospital cardiac arrest - a new early marker of favorable outcome? Resuscitation. 2015;**89**:36-42. DOI: 10.1016/j.resuscitation.2014.12.031

[72] Thomsen JH, Nielsen N, Hassager C, Wanscher M, Pehrson S, Kober L, et al. Bradycardia during targeted temperature management: An early marker of lower mortality and favorable neurologic outcome in comatose out-of-hospital cardiac arrest patients. Critical Care Medicine. 2016;**44**(2):308-318. Epub 2015/10/16. DOI: 10.1097/CCM.0000000000001390

[73] Muengtaweepongsa S, Jantanukul A, Suwanprasert K. Should the heart rate including the heart rate variability be important prognostigators in cardiac arrest? Resuscitation.

2016;**98**:e15. Epub 2015/11/26. DOI: 10.1016/j.resuscitation.2015.08.026

[74] Mejía-Mejía E, Budidha K, Abay TY, May JM, Kyriacou PA. Heart rate variability (HRV) and pulse rate variability (PRV) for the assessment of autonomic responses. Frontiers in Physiology. 2020;**11**:779. DOI: 10.3389/fphys.2020.00779

[75] Jantanukul A, Muengtaweepongsa S, Suwanprasert K, editors. Suppression of autonomic drive determined by nonlinear HRV analysis in therapeutic hypothermia after cardiac arrest. The 6th 2013 Biomedical Engineering International Conference Krabi. IEEE; 2013. DOI: 10.1109/bmeicon.2013.6687657

[76] Kovacs E, Pilecky D, Szakal-Toth Z, Fekete-Gyor A, Gyarmathy VA, Geller L, et al. The role of age in post-cardiac arrest therapy in an elderly patient population. Physiology International. 2020;**107**(2):319-336. Epub 2020/07/22. DOI: 10.1556/2060.2020.00027

[77] Kovacs E, Gyarmathy VA, Pilecky D, Fekete-Gyor A, Szakal-Toth Z, Geller L, et al. An interaction effect analysis of thermodilution-guided hemodynamic optimization, patient condition, and mortality after successful cardiopulmonary resuscitation. International Journal of Environmental Research and Public Health. 2021;**18**(10):5223. Epub 2021/06/03. DOI: 10.3390/ijerph18105223